Gynaecological Endocrinology

Gynaecological Endocrinology

A Guide to Understanding and Management

Maureen Dalton
Consultant in Obstetrics and Gynaecology
Sunderland Area Health Authority
Tyne and Wear, UK

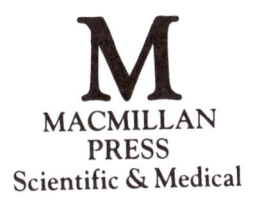

MACMILLAN
PRESS
Scientific & Medical

© Maureen Dalton, 1989
Illustrations © St James's University Hospital, Leeds 1989

All rights reserved. No reproduction, copy or transmission of this publication may be made without written permission.

No paragraph of this publication may be reproduced, copied or transmitted save with written permission or in accordance with the provisions of the Copyright Act 1956 (as amended), or under the terms of any licence permitting limited copying issued by the Copyright Licensing Agency, 33–4 Alfred Place, London WC1E 7DP.

Any person who does any unauthorised act in relation to this publication may be liable to criminal prosecution and civil claims for damages.

First published 1989

Published by
THE MACMILLAN PRESS LTD
Houndmills, Basingstoke, Hampshire RG21 2XS
and London
Companies and representatives
throughout the world

Printed in the People's Republic of China

Typeset by Gecko Limited, Bicester, Oxon

ISBN 0–333–47430–9 (hard cover)
      0–333–47492–9 (paper cover)

Contents

Preface vi
Introduction viii

1	The Hypothalamus	1
2	The Pituitary Gland	5
3	The Gonads	9
4	The Thyroid and Adrenal Glands	12
5	Endorphins and Prostaglandins	19
6	Fat	21
7	Mechanisms of Hormone Action	23
8	Steroid Biochemistry	27
9	Investigations	32
10	The Normal Menstrual Cycle	37
11	Puberty	43
12	The Breast	53
13	Amenorrhoea	57
14	Excessive Menstruation	67
15	Dysmenorrhoea	74
16	Hirsutism	77
17	The Premenstrual Syndrome	84
18	Infertility	91
19	Fertility Control	101
20	Endocrinology of Pregnancy	109
21	The Menopause	114
22	Drugs Used in Gynaecological Endocrinology	120

Bibliography 130
Index 131

Preface

This book has been written to help junior doctors, many of whom have confided in me that they dreaded the gynaecology clinic because they never knew what they could do for the follow-up patient with endocrinological problems, leaving them with a sense of unease about the management of such patients.

Inevitably there will be many who will criticize the book, claiming that too much has been left out or too much put in, and that I have not mentioned their favourite drug or theory. But this guide was not written for those with extensive knowledge of the subject, but for SHOs and others who need the help this book aims to provide.

Theories change and knowledge will eventually change some of the views now held in this rapidly developing field, but the reader will inevitably develop his own reference works as his knowledge and experience grow. Suitable starting works are included in the Bibliography.

There is some deliberate duplication, as it is intended that the book can be 'dipped into' as required and will not necessarily be read from cover to cover. However it is my hope that it will provide for the SHOs and other doctors a useful guide to the understanding and management of the gynaecological patient with endocrinological problems.

I am grateful to Mr Hamish Macdonald, John Barratt, Kate Guthrie and Kaly Bhabra for reading and criticizing the manuscript. Without their hard work this would definitely have been a less complete book. My sincere gratitude also to St James's Hospital Leeds Medical Illustration Department and in particular to Mr Bryan Emmison for his hard work in producing the wonderful illustrations. Thanks also go to Mr David Grist and Mr Richard Powell at The Macmillan Press for their patience, time and guidance, and to David, Sarah and Jennie Holton for their help with the index.

I must also express my special thanks to my parents for their untiring help and encouragement and, finally, but most importantly, to my sister Wendy, who had the unenviable task of translating my indecipherable scribbling into the semblance of a manuscript.

To all of you — thank you.

Leeds, 1989 M.D.

Introduction

This book is not designed to be read from cover to cover. It is meant to be a guide for those who are uncertain about how to manage the diseases described here. Gynaecological endocrinology is a subject where rapid changes are made. This leaves many worried that the subject, which they never really understood as a student, has changed too rapidly. The first section provides a refresher of the physiology, especially aspects such as steroid biochemistry and hormone action which tend to be forgotten by the stage the SHO needs to understand them. The clinical chapters employ tables, figures and flow diagrams as it is hoped that they will help the reader to use the book as a practical guide. For this reason the same picture of a woman has been used repeatedly in figures with overdrawing of the salient features. Those with a pictorial memory will start to remember the aspects to look for in, for example, the examination of hirsutism or menorrhagia from these pictures.

The chapters in the clinical section are arranged in an approximate order of chronological age, from menarche to menopause. They cover the common problems. The starting point in each case is the presenting complaint, e.g. menorrhagia or dysmenorrhoea rather than the common diseases. Thus endometriosis or hypothyroidism will be discussed in more than one chapter. However patients do not present with a tag stating the disease, rather with symptoms. The causes, relevant points of the history and examination, investigations and possible methods of treatment are then covered.

It is hoped that using the diagram of the same woman each time will help to reinforce that the patient should be seen as a whole and that the clues to the answer to the problem do not always lie within the pelvis.

1

The Hypothalamus

INTRODUCTION

The hypothalamus lies in the base of the brain around the floor of the third ventricle, in the area between the optic chiasma and the mammillary bodies. It contains many nuclear groups (see Figure 1.1) including:

1. Paraventricular nuclei
2. Supraoptic nuclei
3. Ventromedial nuclei
4. Median eminence.

The median eminence is connected to the pituitary gland by the pituitary stalk. The nuclei at the base of the hypothalamus produce the releasing and inhibitory hormones, which are involved in the control of the pituitary. The efferent nerve fibres join the hypothalamoneurohypophyseal tract to end in the mass of capillaries known as the 'portal system' of the pituitary. Thus the hypothalamus transforms neural transmission to hormone release at the pituitary. Specialized ciliated cells in the median eminence; called tanycytes, monitor the state of the cerebrospinal fluid (CSF) in the third ventricle.

HORMONES OF THE HYPOTHALAMUS

Table 1.1 lists the hypothalamic hormones and their functions.

Gonadotrophin Releasing Hormone

Gonadotrophin releasing hormone (GnRH) is a decapeptide which releases both follicle stimulating hormone (FSH) and luteinizing hormone (LH). It was originally referred to as the

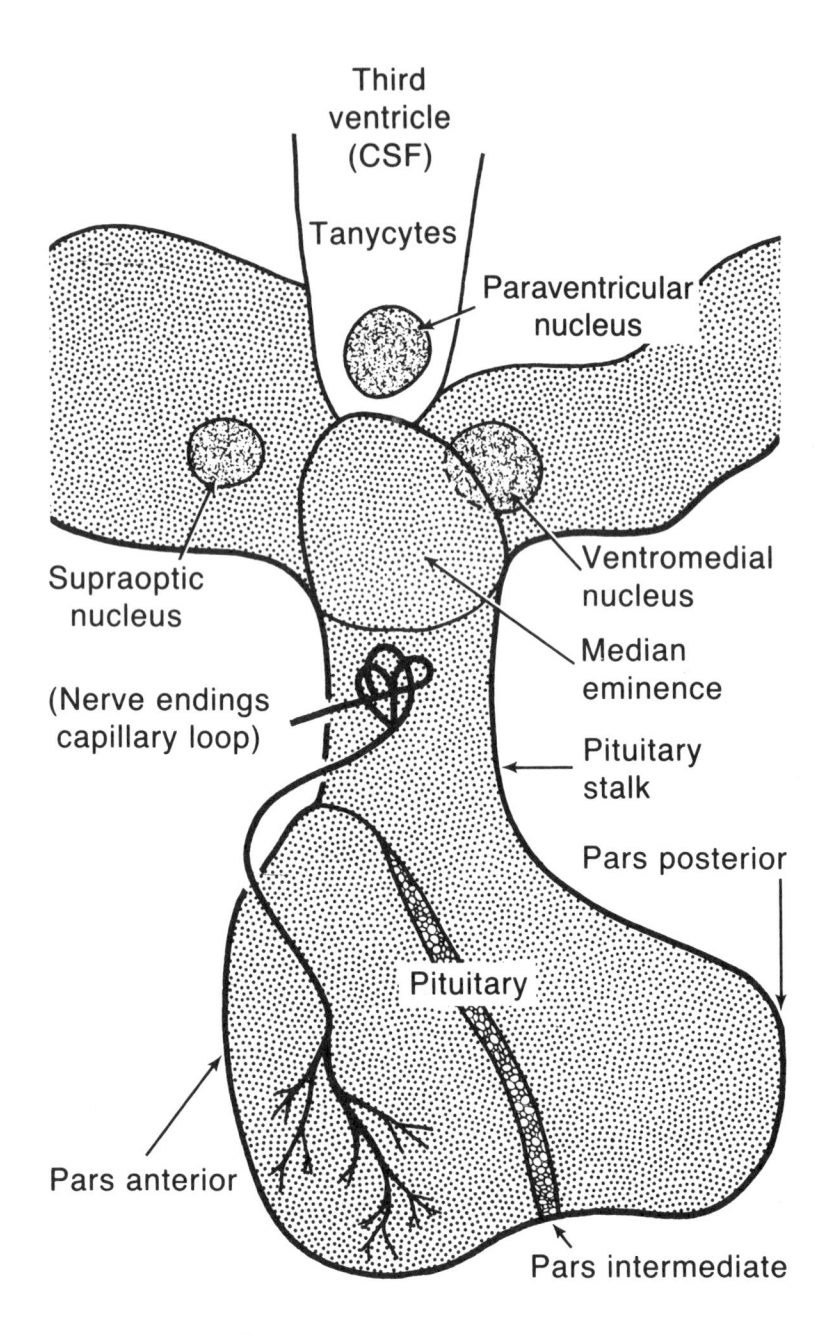

Figure 1.1 The hypothalamus.

The Hypothalamus

luteinizing hormone releasing hormone (LHRH) but it is now recognized as GnRH. It is found in highest concentrations in the lateral pallisade zones of the median eminence, where it is stored as granules in the nerve endings. GnRH is secreted in pulses against a background of continuous low level secretion.

CONTROL

Hypothalamic release is controlled by:

1. Higher neurological centres.
2. Neurotransmitters such as dopamine.
3. Negative feedback from target organs (e.g. FSH and LH from the pituitary, oestradiol and progesterone from the ovary).
4. Ultra-short feedback (see page 25).

Thyrotrophin Releasing Hormone

Thyrotrophin releasing hormone (TRH) is a tripeptide which regulates the release of thyroid stimulating hormone (TSH) from the pituitary. It can also stimulate prolactin (PRL) release.

Somatostatin

Somatostatin is a 14 amino acid peptide which inhibits the release of growth hormone, prolactin, and thyroid stimulating hormone (TSH). It is also found in the intestine, and is involved in insulin metabolism and possibly in pain transmission.

Corticotrophin Releasing Hormone

Corticotrophin releasing hormone (CRH) is a larger peptide containing 41 amino acids. It stimulates secretion of adrenocorticotrophic hormone (ACTH), β lipotrophin and melanocyte stimulating hormone releasing hormone (MSHRH).

THE PINEAL GLAND

The pineal gland is situated on the floor of the third ventricle. Soon after birth it loses its neural connections and develops sympathetic innervation. It appears to respond to photic and hormonal stimuli, and circadian rhythms, and it may have an inhibitory effect on the hypothalamus. The pineal gland can also convert testosterone and progesterone to their five metabolites and aromatize androgens to oestrogens. Tumours of the pineal gland are associated with precocious puberty.

Table 1.1 The hypothalamic stimulating hormones

Hormone	Stimulates
GnRH	FSH
	LH
TRH	TSH
	PRL
CRH	ACTH
	β Lipotrophin
	MSHRH

2

The Pituitary Gland

INTRODUCTION

The pituitary gland is situated in the sella turcica in the base of the skull. It consists of an anterior and a posterior lobe, which can be distinguished anatomically and which have different functions. It receives its blood supply from both the hypothalamus, via the portal system, and the internal carotid artery, via the superior pituitary artery. The cells of the anterior pituitary are surrounded by sinusoids.

THE ANTERIOR PITUITARY

The anterior pituitary contains three types of cells, which can be differentiated by their ability to take up histological stains. They are:

1. *Acidophils*, which form 37% of the total cells and secrete prolactin and growth hormone.
2. *Basophils*, which represent 11% of the total cells and secrete ACTH, TSH, FSH, LH and lipotrophin.
3. *Chromophobe cells*, which form the remaining 52% and may represent exhausted basophils.

The hypothalamus and the pituitary are responsible for the interaction of the hormonal and neural regulation of the reproductive system. The multiple inhibitory and stimulating factors from the hypothalamus interpret the neural stimuli and control pituitary hormone release (Table 2.1). The feedback mechanisms of the pituitary provide sensitive control of the hypothalamus, enabling integrated, appropriate secretion of hormones to occur.

Follicle Stimulating Hormone

Follicle stimulating hormone (FSH) is a glycoprotein and, like LH

(see below), is composed of two subunits, α and β. It has a molecular weight of about 32 000 daltons. Its half-life is about 40 minutes, which is twice as long as that of LH.
Action is to initiate the development of follicles in the ovary.
Control of secretion is by:

1. GnRH released in pulses. A reduction in the frequency of pulses causes an *increase* in FSH.
2. The negative feedback effect of oestradiol.
3. The negative feedback effects of progesterone and testosterone, which also influence GnRH secretion.

Luteinizing Hormone

Luteinizing hormone (LH) is also a glycoprotein composed of two subunits, which differ from FSH only in the subunit; TSH and HCG also share the common subunit. The molecular weight is 28 000 daltons.
Action is to allow the release of the ovum from the follicle of the corpus luteum, and stimulate steroidogenesis in the ovarian stroma.
Control of secretion is by:

1. Large amplitude pulses of GnRH which increase LH. It is seen at night in the prepubertal child. LH tends to be stored as granules so that the massive mid-cycle surge can occur.
2. Increasing oestrogen levels, as found at mid-cycle, exert a positive feedback effect.
3. Negative feedback effect of progesterone.

Prolactin

Prolactin (PRL) is a non-carbohydrate protein with a molecular weight of 24 000 daltons. Its structure is similar to growth hormone and human placental lactogen.
Action is to stimulate the differentiation and growth of breast tissue and maintain milk secretion. In excess, it is able to block the action of FSH and LH.
Control is suggested by recent evidence that prolactin secretion is inhibited via dopamine and gonadotrophin-associated protein (GAP) which is a peptide on the GnRH prohormone. Prolactin is stimulated by two hormones, vasoactive intestinal protein (VIP) and peptide histidine isoleucine (PHI), which are both found on the same prohormone. They represent prolactin inhibitory factor (PIF) and prolactin releasing factor (PRF), respectively.

Table 2.1 Pituitary control

Stimulates	Inhibits
GnRH → FSH, LH	GAP
VIP → PRL	Dopamine → PRL
PHI → PRL	
TRH → PRL, TSH	Somatostatin → TSH, GH
GNRH → GH	

| Vasopressin → ACTH | |
| CRH → ACTH, β endorphin, β lipotrophin | |

Adrenocorticotrophin

Adrenocorticotrophin (ACTH) is derived from pro-opiomelanocortin, which splits to form MSH and corticotrophic intermediate lobe protein (CLIP), endorphin and metakephalin, as well as ACTH. It is a polypeptide of 39 amino acids with a molecular weight of 4500 daltons.
Action is to stimulate the adrenal cortex to synthesize cortisol. It has a diurnal rhythm of secretion.
Control is by negative feedback of cortisol on CRH.

THE POSTERIOR PITUITARY

The posterior pituitary secretes vasopressin, oxytocin and neurophysin. They are synthesized in the supraoptic and paraventricular nuclei and transported down the axons of the neurohypophyseal tract.

Vasopressin

Vasopressin is a nonapeptide with a molecular weight of 1000 daltons.

Action is on the distal tubules and collecting ducts of the kidney. *Control* involves the osmolarity of plasma and plasma volume. It was formerly known as antidiuretic hormone (ADH).

Oxytocin

Oxytocin is also a nonapeptide and only differs from vasopressin by one amino acid molecule, which accounts for some of the overlap in function. It also has a molecular weight of 1000 daltons. *Action* is to stimulate uterine activity, although it also has a mild antidiuretic action. It is involved in the ejection of milk and may also be involved in the maturation of the ovum.

3

The Gonads

THE OVARIES

There are two hormone producing compartments in the ovary:
1. The follicle and corpus luteum
2. The ovarian stroma.

The main hormones produced by the ovaries are *oestradiol, progesterone* and *androstenedione*, which is secreted mainly by the stroma and is converted to other steroids in the fat.

Oestrogens

Oestradiol (E2) is the major hormone of the ovary and is produced by the follicle throughout the menstrual cycle in varying amounts, the highest levels occurring in the follicular phase.

Oestrone (E1) is the main oestrogen found in postmenopausal women; it mainly comes from conversion of androstenedione.

Oestriol (E3) is found in high levels in pregnancy. It is converted from oestradiol and oestrone and is much weaker in its action.

The major actions are:

1. The maintenance of secondary sexual characteristics.
2. The development of the female breast.
3. The laying down of fat in the female distribution.
4. Vulval and vaginal hypertrophy.
5. Proliferation of the endometrium (see page 40).
6. Maturation of the oocyte.
7. Calcification of bone.
8. Increase in production of binding protein.
9. Increase in factors VII, VIII, IX and X for blood clotting.
10. Inhibition of conversion of tryptophan to serotonin.

Oestradiol production is controlled by the negative feeback effect of FSH. It is bound in the blood to sex hormone binding globulin (SHBG) and albumin, and is metabolized by the liver.

Progesterone

Progesterone is produced in large quantities in the corpus luteum. It is also produced by the adrenal glands where it holds a key position in the steroid pathway, many steroids being produced by changes from progesterone (see page 29).
Its actions are:

1. Induction of 'secretory' changes in the endometrium (see page 41).
2. Thickening of cervical mucus, making it appear opaque.
3. Induction of changes in uterine contractions.
4. Relaxation of smooth muscle.
5. Stimulation of glandular development in the breast.
6. Increase body temperature.
7. Antagonization of aldosterone.
8. Antihypertensive effects.
9. Increase respiratory volume and reduce pCO_2.
10. Bound in plasma to cortisol binding globulin.

Progesterone production in the corpus luteum is affected by LH and in the adrenal glands by ACTH.

Androstenedione

Androstenedione is produced by the theca cells and the stroma. LH stimulates its production. It is weakly androgenic and can be converted into testosterone and oestrone.

Inhibin

Inhibin is a protein with a molecular weight of 71 000 daltons found in follicular fluid. It inhibits FSH release by negative feedback. It is also present in the testes.

THE TESTES

The testes are concerned with the production of sperm and the androgens.
Testosterone is the major androgen produced in the testes, but *dihydrotestosterone (DHT), 4-androstendione* and *dehydroepi-*

androsterone are also produced in the testes, together with a very small amount of *oestrogen*.

The control of steroidogenesis in the testes is by LH via a negative feedback mechanism. LH, FSH and the androgens produced in the testes are required for spermatogenesis. *Inhibin* is produced by the testes and is involved in spermatogenesis; it exerts a feedback effect on FSH release.

4

The Thyroid and Adrenal Glands

THE THYROID GLAND

The thyroid gland consists of two lobes joined by a central band. It iodinates tyrosine to produce thyroxine (T4) and tri-iodothyronine (T3).
 T4 is bound in the plasma to:
1. thyroxine binding globulin (TBG),
2. thyroxine binding pre-albumin (TBPA),
3. albumin.

T3 binds with less affinity to TBG and *not* to TBPA. T4 can be converted into T3 in the peripheral tissues. T3 is much more potent than T4 which is relatively inactive. T3 and T4 are also conjugated in the liver.

Actions of Tri-iodothyronine

1. Control of the basal metabolic rate, including oxygen consumption and heat control.
2. Stimulation of normal growth.
3. Stimulation of muscle contractions.
4. Stimulation of lipid formation and lipolysis.
5. Stimulation of enzyme synthesis.

The thyroid hormones and their actions are outlined in Table 4.1. The mechanisms of action are unknown.

Control of Thyroxine Release

T4 release is controlled by TSH, which in turn is controlled by a negative feedback of T4 on the pituitary. Thus, measurement of TSH is a sensitive approximate guide to thyroid function; it is low in hyperthyroidism, absent in secondary hypothyroidism and raised in primary hypothyroidism.

The Thyroid and Adrenal Glands

Table 4.1 The thyroid hormones

Hormone	Action	Control
Thyroxine T4	Converted to T3 in peripheral tissues	TSH — negative feedback
Tri-iodothyronine T3	Control of basal metabolites	TSH
	Stimulation of lipid formation and lipolysis	
	Stimulation of enzyme synthesis	
Calcitonin	Reduction of plasma Ca^{2+}	Serum Ca^{2+} levels?
	Inhibition of bone resorption	

Calcitonin

This is a polypeptide with a molecular weight of 3000 daltons. It is secreted by the parafollicular cells (C cells) of the thyroid, under the control of the parathyroid hormone (parathormone).

Action is to reduce plasma calcium by inhibition of bone resorption.
Control is by serum calcium levels.

Parathyroid Glands

The parathyroid glands are situated just posterior to the thyroid gland. There are usually four glands, but they can vary in number from two to six. They secrete *parathormone*, which is a polypeptide involved in calcium metabolism. The parathormone levels rise as plasma calcium levels fall.

Calcium Metabolism

In an average western diet, 25 mmol of calcium are consumed each day, of which 4 mmol are absorbed and the rest excreted in the faeces. The absorption of calcium occurs in the small intestine.

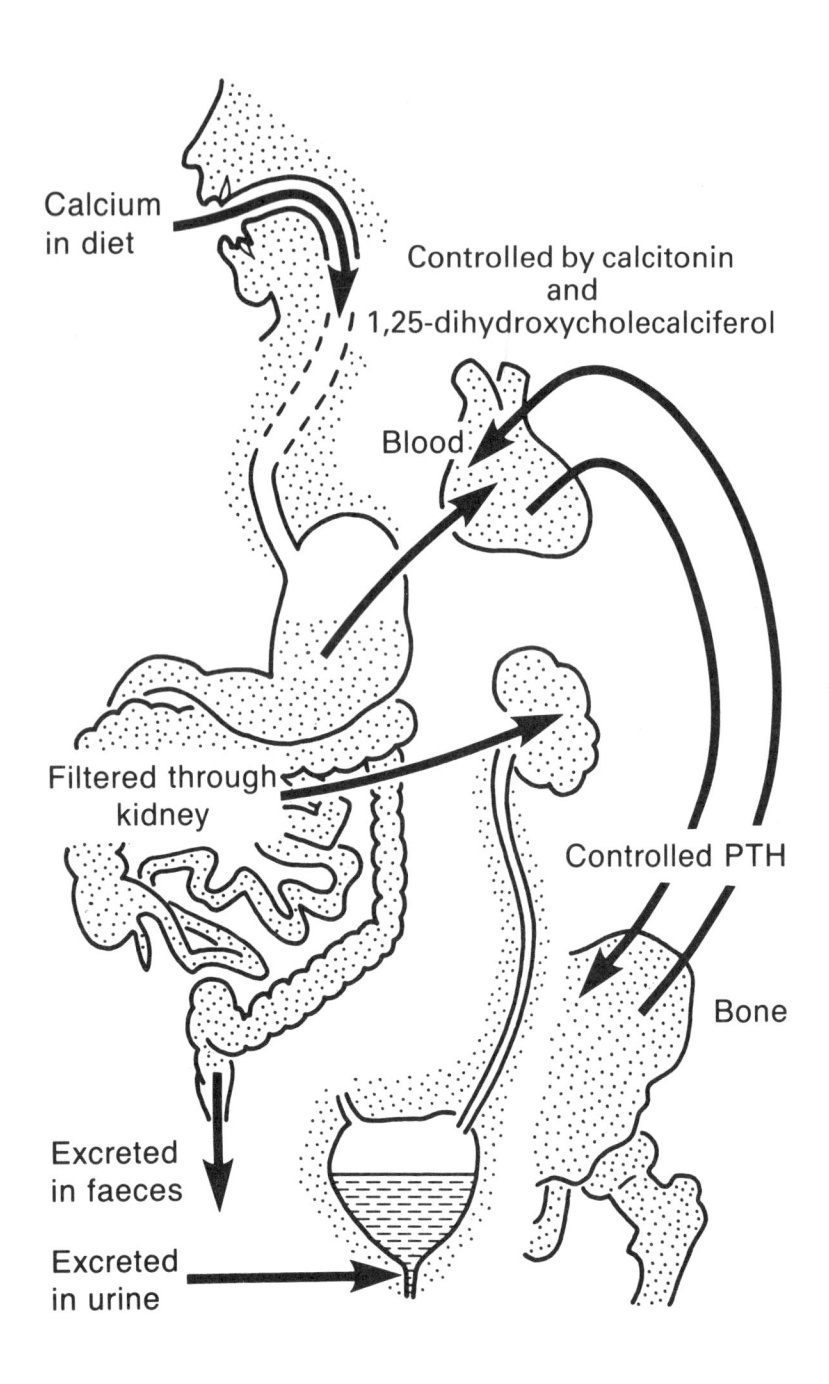

Figure 4.1 Metabolism of calcium.

Each day 175 mmol of calcium is filtered through the kidneys, the vast majority being resorbed with only about 5 mmol being excreted. Calcium is also being continuously mobilized and deposited in the bone (see Figure 4.1).

The range for plasma calcium levels is limited as calcium metabolism is kept under very close control. Control is principally maintained by:

1. Parathormone
2. Calcitonin
3. 1,25-Dihydroxycholecalciferol.

1,25-Dihydroxycholecalciferol is a metabolite of vitamin D which is hydroxylated first in the liver and then transported in the plasma to the kidney where it is further hydroxylated. It is needed for the active transport of calcium in the small intestine.

THE ADRENAL GLANDS

The two adrenal glands are composed of cortex and medulla, which have different embryological origins. They are situated above the kidneys and are pyramidal in shape.

Adrenal Cortex

The adrenal cortex is composed of three layers:

1. The zona glomerulosa which synthesizes the mineralocorticoids (i.e. aldosterone).
2. The zona fasciculata which synthesizes the corticosteroids (e.g. cortisol).
3. The zona reticularis which synthesizes androgens and to a lesser extent oestrogens.

The action and control of the hormones is given in Table 4.2.

MINERALOCORTICOSTEROIDS

Aldosterone is the main mineralocorticoid; its action is to increase sodium absorption from the distal tubule and the loops of Henle. Its control is via the renin-angiotensin system.

Table 4.2 Hormones of the adrenal cortex

Layer	Hormones	Action	Control
Zona glomerulosa	Mineralocorticoids (aldosterone)	Increasing sodium absorption from distal tubules	Renin-angiotensin system
Zona fasciculata	Corticosteroids (cortisone and corticosterone)	Enhancing gluconeogenesis Protein catabolism Fat deposition Insulin antagonist Anti-inflammatory Immunosuppression Decreasing host immune response	Negative feedback from ACTH
Zona reticularis	Androgens (testosterone, androstenedione and dehydroepiandrosterone)	Masculinization Anabolic Stimulation of cell growth Increasing muscle mass and bodyweight	ACTH

GLUCOCORTICOSTEROIDS

Cortisone and corticosterone are the commonest examples of this group of steroids.
Actions:

1. Enhancing gluconeogenesis.
2. Protein catabolism.
3. Fat disposition on the face, neck and trunk.
4. Peripheral antagonism to insulin.
5. Anti-inflammatory actions, e.g. decreasing host response to infection.
6. Immunosuppressive actions, e.g. decreasing antibody production.
7. Involvement in delayed hypersensitivity.

Secretion is controlled by negative feedback of ACTH. Cortisol is bound in the blood to cortisol binding globulin (CBG).

ANDROGENS

Dehydroepiandrosterone, testosterone and androstenedione are the commonest androgens.
Actions:

1. Masculinization.
2. Anabolic.
3. Stimulating cell growth.
4. Increasing muscle mass and body weight.

Adrenal Medulla

The adrenal medulla is composed of chromaffin cells which arise embryologically from the neural crest. They secrete adrenalin, which is converted by the adrenal medulla from noradrenalin. There are two types of adrenergic receptors, α and β.

α RECEPTORS

The α receptors respond by causing vasoconstriction.

β RECEPTORS
Actions:

1. Dilate arteries.

2. Increase heart rate.
3. Increase atrial and ventricular contractility and conduction rate.
4. Dilate bronchioles.
5. Increase blood glucose.

5

Endorphins and Prostaglandins

ENDORPHINS

Endorphins are peptides found in the brain that bind to opioid receptors. Pro-opiomelanocortin (see page 26) splits to produce enkephalin, α-lipotrophin (αLPH) and endorphins.
Proposed actions include:
1. The modification of perception of pain.
2. The regulation of temperature and satiety.
3. Inhibition of LH, FSH, ACTH and TSH.
4. Stimulation of prolactin and growth hormone.
5. Inhibition of vasopressin and oxytocin.

Endorphins may be implicated in some cases of amenorrhoea, particularly exercise-induced amenorrhoea, and possibly also in the premenstrual syndrome.

PROSTAGLANDINS

The prostaglandins (PG) are a large group of compounds made from fatty acid precursors. They were originally found in seminal fluid and are found in many tissues in the body. The most important prostaglandins in reproductive physiology are derived from arachnodonic acid and belong to the PG2 group of compounds. In our present state of knowledge, the two prostaglandins most relevant in reproduction are $PGF_2\alpha$ and PGE_2. Other prostaglandins, *thromboxane* and *prostacyclin* (PG1), have opposing actions on platelets and blood vessels and may be relevant in endometrial shedding and pre-eclampsia. They are metabolized very rapidly, making investigation into their role more difficult.

Actions

PGF$_2\alpha$ induces rupture of the ovarian follicle by an anti-LH action. High doses of oestrogen can stimulate PGF$_2\alpha$ and thus induce ovarian follicle rupture, which may account for the ability of high doses of oestrogen to act as a post-coital contraception.

In some species PGF$_2\alpha$ causes luteal regression if implantation has not occurred. PGF$_2\alpha$ and PGE$_2$ both cause contraction of the non-pregnant and pregnant uterus when administered intravenously.

In the fetus the patency of the ductus arteriosus appears to depend on PGE$_2$. PG synthetase inhibitors can successfully close persistent patent ductus arteriosus after delivery in about 40% of cases.

6

Fat

INTRODUCTION

Fat is an endocrine organ with the ability to convert steroids to produce *androgens* and *oestrogens*. It is not under the simple control of FSH and LH and so may produce oestrogens inappropriately. Thus, fat has many gynaecological effects.

BIOCHEMISTRY

The body fat can convert androstenedione to *testosterone, oestradiol* and *oestrone*. The mechanisms involved are not fully understood, but oestrogen production in fat is related to a certain degree to the extent of obesity. In addition, sex hormone binding globulin is low in obese people, resulting in an even greater increase in the free oestradiol.

OBESITY

Causes

1. Idiopathic.
2. Neurological (lesions in the ventromedial nucleus).
3. Genetic predisposition.
4. Endocrine
    (a) hypothyroidism
    (b) Cushing's syndrome
    (c) acromegaly
    (d) polycystic ovary syndrome (PCO).

Endocrinological Complications

Due to increased testosterone:

1. Hirsutism

Due to increased oestrogen:

1. Amenorrhoea
2. Anovulation (heavy or irregular periods)
3. Endometrial hyperplasia and endometrial carcinoma
4. Polycystic ovary syndrome.

7

Mechanisms of Hormone Action

INTRODUCTION

Definition
    Hormones are chemical signals in a complex internal biological communication system. They are secreted at one site and act at another site.

Hormones play a vital role in the male and female, in every facet of reproduction. Consequently gynaecologists spend a considerable amount of time diagnosing and treating hormonal dysfunction.

Modes of Dysfunction

1. Inappropriate secretion of a hormone or hormones by an organ, e.g. overproduction of prolactin by the pituitary causing amenorrhoea, underproduction of thyroid hormones causing amenorrhoea and dysfunctional uterine bleeding.
2. Inappropriate reception of the hormonal stimulus by the target tissue, e.g. resistant ovary syndrome, in which the ovary cannot respond to FSH.

Reproductive hormones bind to specific receptors. There are two main classes of hormones involved in reproduction:

1. The *peptide hormones*, e.g. FSH, LH, GnRH and prolactin.
2. The *steroid hormones*, e.g. testosterone, oestradiol and progesterone.

PEPTIDE HORMONES

The peptide hormones pass messages and tend to remain on the surface of the cell. In order to induce a response within the cell, an enzyme called cyclic adenosine monophosphate (cAMP) is used as a second messenger. cAMP binds to protein kinase which can then phosphorylate various proteins, thus enabling the peptide hormone to induce changes in the endocrine environment; for example, the protein may increase the steroid production.

STEROID HORMONES

The steroid hormones have a different mechanism of action. They are able to diffuse into cells because they are so much smaller. In the circulation they are loosely bound to albumin and more specifically to special binding proteins.

Dihydrotestosterone (DHT), testosterone (T) and oestradiol (E_2) bind to sex hormone binding globulin (SHBG) which is also known as testosterone oestradiol binding globulin (TeBG). Progesterone and cortisol are bound to cortisol binding globulin (CBG). The question of whether the steroid is biologically inactive while bound to a binding protein has recently been raised. There is evidence to suggest that at some sites of action it is the bound steroid that is the active fraction, while at other sites the unbound or free steroid is the active fraction binding to the receptor on the cell wall. The complete mechanism of action of the steroid binding proteins has not been completely clarified, although much research is in progress.

Once bound to a receptor, the steroid can then move into the cell. It will be translocated to the nucleus to interact with the receptor site on the genome; this allows synthesis of RNA, directing the amino acid sequence of a new protein. Testosterone is usually converted to DHT in the cell before it binds on to the genome.

Some hormones do not fall into either of these categories, e.g. thyroxine, prostaglandins.

HORMONAL FEEDBACK

Negative Feedback

This occurs when the high concentration of one hormone results in a reduction of the hormone that stimulates its production. For example, high oestradiol reduces FSH and high progesterone reduces LH.

Positive Feedback

This occurs when the concentration of one hormone results in an increase of the hormone that stimulates its production. For example, oestradiol stimulation of LH at ovulation.

Long Feedback

This is the loop of feedback of control from the target organ to the pituitary and hypothalamus. For example, oestradiol control of GnRH release.

Short Feedback

This is the effect of the pituitary hormone on the release of its hypothalamic releasing factors. For example, the effect of FSH release on GnRH.

Ultrashort Feedback

This is the effect of the release of a hypothalamic hormone on its own release by influencing storage and manufacture. For example, GnRH affecting GnRH release which leads to pulsatility of GnRH release.

SECRETION

Some hormones are synthesized in the gland and immediately secreted into the circulation, e.g. ovarian oestradiol production. Other hormones are synthesized and stored until the appropriate stimulus for release occurs, e.g. thyroxine in the thyroid gland or LH from the pituitary. Hormones which are stored and then secreted can be released in pulses. The amplitude and the frequency of these pulses may be critical to the effect caused. Increasing the pulse frequency of GnRH within a narrow range decreases LH release and increases FSH release.

Hormones that are stored may be manufactured in a different area from where they are released, e.g. vasopressin is synthesized in the hypothalamus and stored in the pituitary.

Hormones may have precursor forms from which some amino acid chains are broken off to release the active hormone, for example, thyroglobulin to thyroxine. This method makes it possible for one protein to produce various hormones, depending on the site of cleavage. The most complex example is probably the hypothalamic hormone *pro-opiomelanocortin*, which can be split first to produce the peptide ACTH intermediate or the peptide β lipotrophin. These can also be split so that eventually the former produces ACTH and the latter melanotrophin stimulating hormone (MSH) which, in turn, form corticotrophin-like intermediate lobe protein (CLIP), the enkephalins and the endorphins.

REGULATION

Up Regulation

Hormones can sometimes influence their own cell membrane receptor production. For example, acidophils increase the number of their own cell receptors and thus become less sensitive to changes in prolactin concentration.

Desensitization or Down Regulation

An excess of a hormone can also sometimes result in a reduction in the number of the cell receptors for that hormone and so lessen the sensitivity to that hormone. The term desensitization is thus a more accurate term for this phenomenon. For example, excess GnRH or analogues of GnRH administered in a constant, as opposed to pulsed rate, reduces the ability of the basophils to respond to GnRH by producing LH and FSH.

8

Steroid Biochemistry

In order to comprehend reproductive endocrinology, it is important to understand the basic differences in some of the steroid hormones. This can be difficult to follow as the chemical structures look very similar. The basic steroid structure is three 6-carbon rings and one 5-carbon ring arranged as shown here. The chemical name is a *perhydrocyclopentaphenantrene ring*.

All the carbon atoms in steroid rings are numbered 1 to 17.

Most of the relevant changes occur at C3 or at C17.

Small changes in structure make great differences in the ability of the molecule to bind to a specific receptor and so affect the mode of action. All steroids are synthesized from *acetate* to *cholesterol* which is then converted to *pregnenolone*. This has a CH_3 radical at C17 and an OH radical at C3.

Cholesterol

Pregnenolone

Pregnenolone can change in two possible ways, called Δ4 and Δ5 pathways. These act as metabolic pathways that the steroids can pass down and so represent two different routes of metabolism.

In the Δ4 pathway, C3 changes from OH to =O and the double bond between C5 and C6 swings round to C4 and C5. This is *progesterone*.

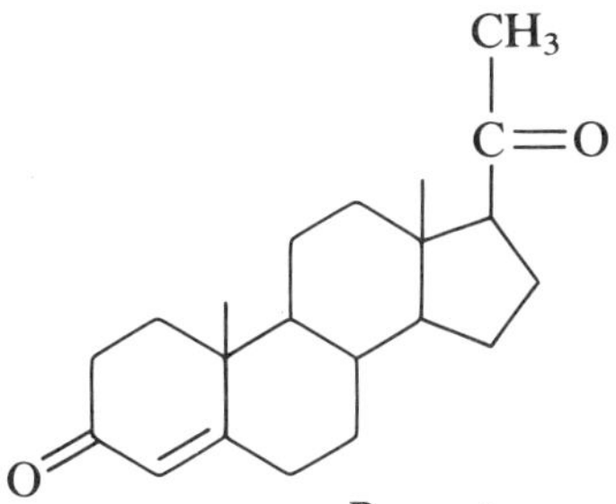

Progesterone

If the CH3 radical at C17 was changed to an OH, this would be *testosterone*. This is a *small* change but it produces *large* differences in action.

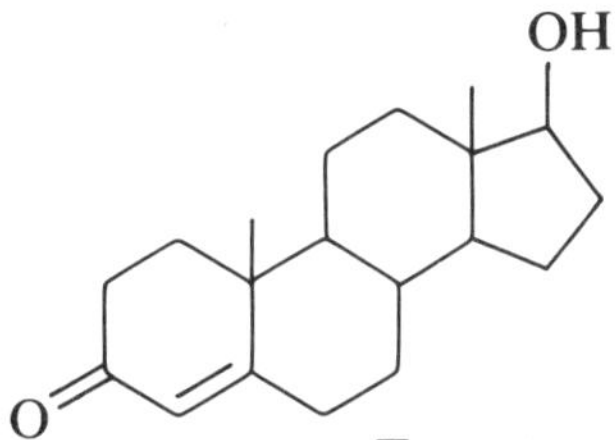

Testosterone

Changing to an OH radical at C3 and reorganizing the double bonds on the first (A) benzene ring produces a hormone with very different actions, *oestradiol*.

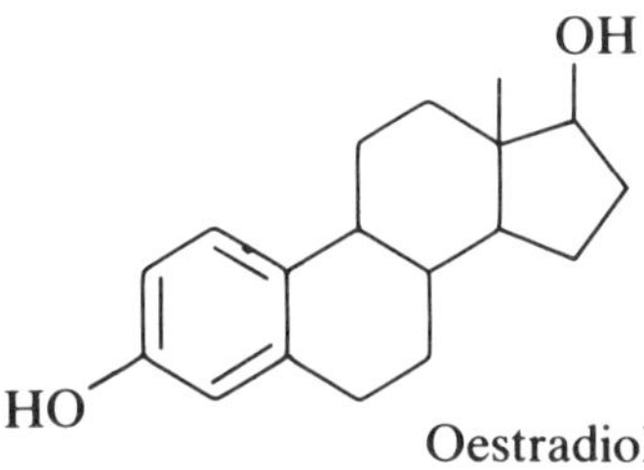

Oestradiol

Reorganizing the double bonds is called aromatization. *Oestrone* only differs at C17, where OH is changed to =O.

Oestrone

This is a Δ 5 steroid, so called because it can be metabolized via the Δ5 enzymatic pathway from pregnenolone.

The steroids are grouped together according to the number of carbon atoms in the molecule. The C21 steroids, for example progesterone, have 21 carbon atoms.

Most *androgens* are C19 steroids.
Most *oestrogens* are C18 steroids.

C19 steroids with an oxygen atom at C17 are sometimes referred to as the *17 oxosteroids* or *17 ketosteroids*. These will be androgenic because they are C19 steroids.

One of the reasons why such small changes in structure can produce such marked differences in action is because of the three-dimensional nature of the molecule. The benzene ring can exist in two forms: the 'boat' and the 'chair'.

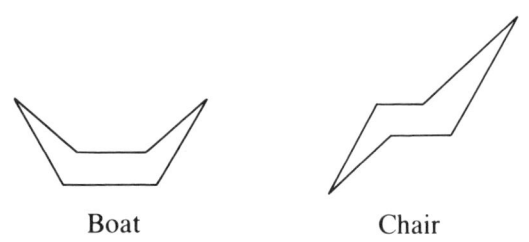

Boat   Chair

When two benzene rings combine, they can join in different ways: two 'chairs' joined together produce the *cis* form; a 'boat' and a 'chair' together make the *trans* form.

Cis

Trans

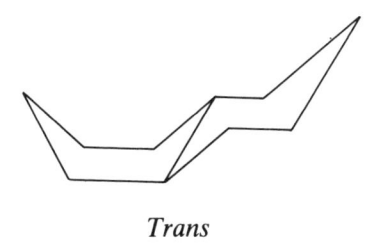

These changes will obviously appear very different to the steroid receptor. The C and D rings are always in the *trans* position, but the A and B rings may be in either the *cis* or *trans* position. Any additional radicals on the molecule can be attached in two different planes, above or below the plane of the benzene ring.

One of the various stages in the enzymatic pathways can occasionally be absent, such as in the various forms of congenital adrenal hyperplasia which is an autosomal recessive condition.

9

Investigations

INTRODUCTION

Investigations used in gynaecological endocrinology can be divided into two broad groups:
1. The observation of a biological effect.
2. The specific quantification of a substance.

OBSERVATION OF A BIOLOGICAL EFFECT

Hormone release by the endocrine glands is controlled by various different stimuli.

Dynamic Testing

If a gland is underfunctioning, it may be because it is lacking in stimulation or because it is reponding to the correct stimulation with its maximum output already. If a known stimulator of that gland is administered and the output closely monitored, the cause of hypofunction may be clarified (Figure 9.1).

For example, GnRH (100 nmol) administered intravenously, with estimations of FSH and LH at 0, 20 and 60 minutes, will differentiate a hypothalamic from a pituitary cause of amenorrhoea. If the cause is hypothalamic the pituitary will respond normally, whereas if there is a pituitary cause then no change will be observed.

The pituitary response to TRH infusion can be even more discriminating (Table 9.1). In hyperthyroidism there is no response because of the overwhelming negative feedback response caused by the excess thyroxine, whereas in euthyroidism the normal response is evoked with a moderate rise in TSH, and in hypothroidism there is an exaggerated response.

Investigations

Faulty ----→ GLAND ----→ **Insufficient**
stimulation   Normal   hormonal output
                 synthesis

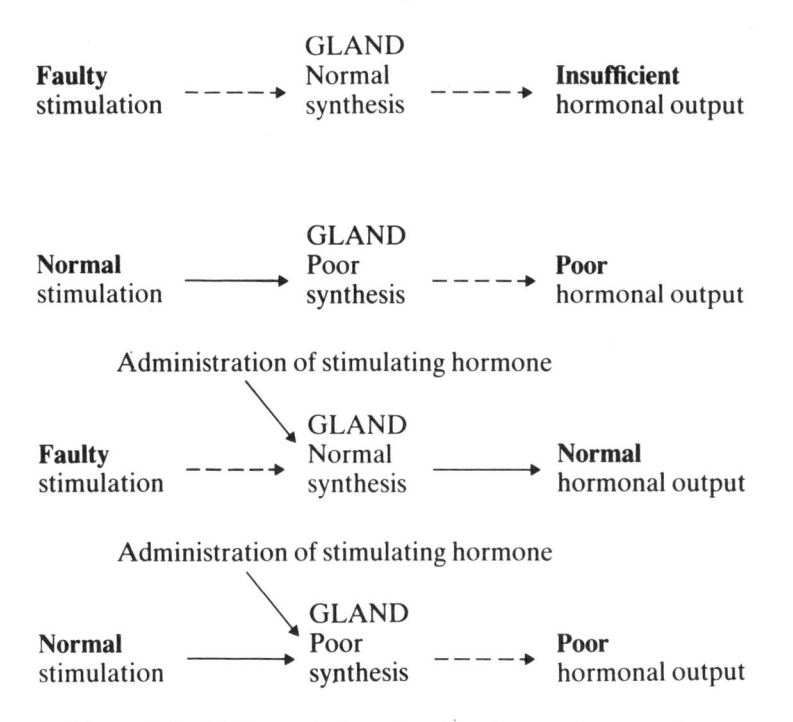

Normal ⟶ GLAND ----→ **Poor**
stimulation   Poor   hormonal output
              synthesis

Administration of stimulating hormone
                    ↘ GLAND
Faulty ----→ Normal ⟶ **Normal**
stimulation   synthesis   hormonal output

Administration of stimulating hormone
                    ↘ GLAND
Normal ⟶ Poor ----→ **Poor**
stimulation   synthesis   hormonal output

Figure 9.1 Differentiation of reduced hormal output due to insufficient stimulation or reduced synthesis.

Table 9.1 Dynamic testing with TRH stimulation

	Pituitary	Thyroid	Response
Hypothalamic TRH ⟶	TSH ⟶	T4	
Hypothalamic TRH plus Exogenous TRH ⟶	TSH ⟶	Hyperthyroid	None
		Euthyroid	Moderate
		Hypothyroid	Excessive

The opposite effect can also be observed (Table 9.2). A normally controlled gland will suppress its hormone release. If the gland is functioning autonomously (as with a tumour), it will not suppress hormone release. For example, in the dexamethasone suppression test, 1 mg is given orally at midnight and the plasma cortisol sample at 8.00 h will be less than $6 \text{g} \text{l}^{-1}$ if the adrenal gland is responding normally. If the adrenal gland has not been suppressed, a longer course of dexamethasone is given and if the adrenal output is still unchanged, Cushing's syndrome or an adrenal tumour must be suspected.

Table 9.2 Dynamic testing by suppression

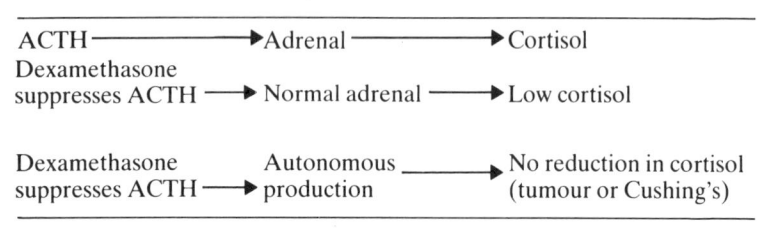

ACTH ⟶	Adrenal ⟶	Cortisol
Dexamethasone suppresses ACTH ⟶	Normal adrenal ⟶	Low cortisol
Dexamethasone suppresses ACTH ⟶	Autonomous production ⟶	No reduction in cortisol (tumour or Cushing's)

Progestogen Challenge Test

A small dose of a progestogen, usually medroxyprogesterone acetate 10 mg b.d. for 5 days, is administered and then stopped. If there is circulating endogenous oestrogen, this will stimulate the endometrium and induce a progestogen withdrawal bleed. This test may be used in amenorrhoeic infertile women.

Daily Ultrasound Scanning

Daily ultrasound scanning is carried out to observe follicular development and confirm the number of follicles ripening, ovulation or the formation of 'luteinized unruptured follicles' (LUFs).

X-ray of the Pituitary Fossa

An x-ray to observe the thinning of the floor of the sella turcica (double floor) is taken whenever a pituitary tumour is suspected. Tomograms or, if appropriate, CAT scans, will visualize the tumour.

SPECIFIC QUANTIFICATION OF A SUBSTANCE

Biological Assays

Biological assays utilize the dose–response measurement of the effect of a hormone on an animal. They are non-specific, time consuming and are now infrequently used. Some years ago, pregnancy tests were performed by observing the ability of toads to produce frogspawn when they were exposed to urine containing high levels of HCG.

Immunoassays

Immunoassays depend on raising an antibody to the substance to be assayed, which must therefore be available in a pure form.

Competitive Protein Binding/Radioimmunoassay (RIA)

These assays work on the principle that the number of binding sites on the antibody raised is limited, therefore a radioactively labelled form of the hormone and the 'naturally occurring' form will compete equally for the binding site. Thus, if there is a large amount of the unlabelled endogenous form in the sample, there will be less opportunity for the labelled hormone to bind to the antibody than if there were very little endogenous hormone. Measuring the radioactivity of the sample and comparing it to an already constructed concentration response curve will allow a concentration of that hormone to be calculated. This assay can be very specific. However, cross-reactivity can occur, for example, many routinely used LH assays cannot distinguish between LH and HCG. However, if an unexpected result is found, the test should be repeated to confirm its accuracy because it is possible for an error to occur.

Binding Assays

The free or unbound fraction of a hormone is the biologically active portion. It is difficult to raise an antibody that can distinguish the free from the bound fraction, particularly as the binding process is a dynamic one in which the bound molecules are changing all the time. Tests to separate the two fractions may rely on a filter that will not allow proteins through, so that separation can occur between the bound and free. Once the sample has reached equilibrium, it is possible to remove the fluid outside the membrane to measure the free fraction. Alternatively, the concentration of the binding protein may be measured and its affinity for the hormone obtained. When adjustments have been made for interaction with other proteins, the level of the free hormone can be calculated. Table 9.3 summarizes the types of investigations used in gynaecological endocrinology.

Table 9.3 Hormonal investigations

Method	Test	Example
Dynamic testing	Stimulating the gland	GnRH, TRH test
	Suppressing hormone release	Dexamethasone suppression test
	Challenge test	Progestogen
	Ultrasound scanning	Ripening of ovarian follicle
Specific quantification	Biological assays	Progestogen potency
	Competitive protein binding	Oestradiol, FSH, LH Thyroxine, progesterone
	Estimation of free hormone	Thyroxine, testosterone

10

The Normal Menstrual Cycle

INTRODUCTION

Menstruation is the result of complex changes in the endometrium under hormonal control and the result of failure to conceive. For regular menstruation to occur, the hypothalamus, pituitary, ovary and uterus must be intact. In a normal menstrual cycle, a follicle must develop, rupture and luteinize. A normal menstrual cycle varies in duration, 24–32 days being the average time from the first day of bleeding to the first day of the next cycle.

THE DEVELOPING FOLLICLE

Each ovarian follicle begins as a primordial follicle, which contains an oocyte (arrested in the meiotic phase) surrounded by a layer of granulosa cells (Figure 10.1). What initiates observed follicular growth is unknown, but it can be observed occurring in the ovary from fetal life until the menopause. The early developing follicle is called a *preantral follicle* and once it has begun to develop it needs FSH stimulation to enable it to continue. The follicle must therefore produce FSH receptors in order to respond to FSH. The FSH receptor will further stimulate the follicle to develop more FSH receptors and FSH in turn will stimulate steroidogenesis. This will increase the oestrogen content of the preantral follicle; the oestrogen content of the follicle is thus limited by the number of FSH receptors. As the number of FSH receptors increases, so the amount of FSH bound to them will increase and, in turn, the oestrogen concentration will increase. Eventually one follicle, the one that started to develop at the optimal time to benefit from the rise in FSH and make the maximum use of its FSH receptors, will develop into the *dominant follicle*. This usually occurs around day 7 of a 28-day cycle. Under normal circumstances only one follicle tends to develop, the others becoming atretic. If exogenous gonadotrophins are given at this stage, it is possible to 'override' this tendency, resulting in more than one follicle developing, thus increasing the chance of multiple births.

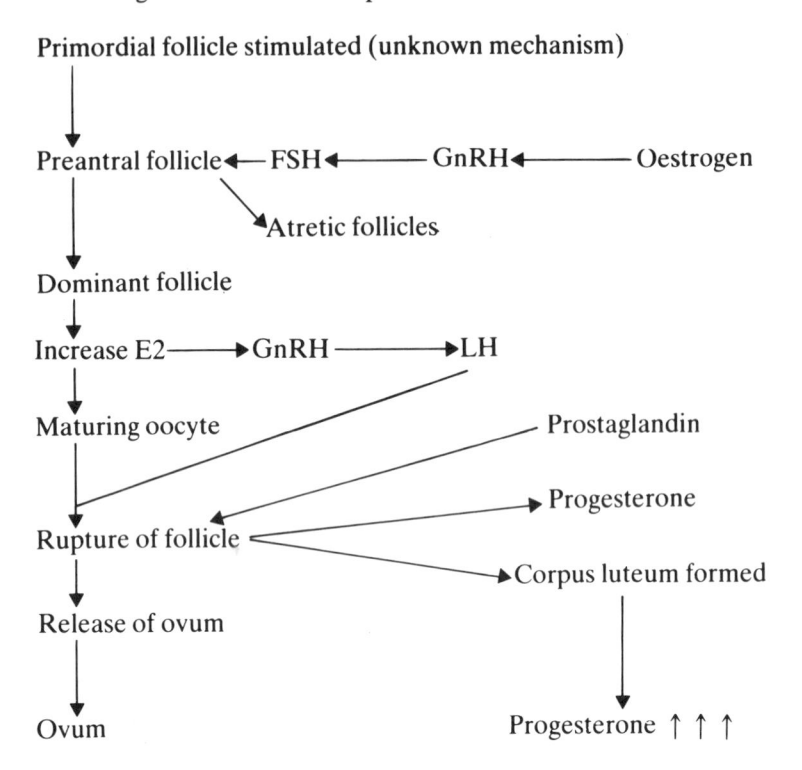

```
Primordial follicle stimulated (unknown mechanism)
        │
        ▼
Preantral follicle ◄─ FSH ◄──── GnRH ◄──── Oestrogen
        │         ↘
        │          Atretic follicles
        ▼
Dominant follicle
        │
        ▼
Increase E2 ────► GnRH ────► LH
        │                    ╲
        ▼                     ╲── Prostaglandin
Maturing oocyte                ╲
        │                       ► Progesterone
        ▼
Rupture of follicle ◄──────────► Corpus luteum formed
        │                              │
        ▼                              ▼
Release of ovum                  Progesterone ↑↑↑
        │
        ▼
Ovum
```

Figure 10.1   Oocyte development.

The dominant follicle continues to develop, and produces large amounts of oestradiol. The presence of high oestradiol and FSH levels stimulates the follicle to make LH receptors. When the follicle has produced enough oestradiol, plasma oestradiol reaches a critical level and the pituitary is stimulated to release LH — the 'LH surge'. There is usually a very small increase in progesterone at this stage, and a sharp fall in oestradiol and FSH. At this time, the maturing oocyte, with its surrounding cells, called the *cumulus* can sometimes be seen by ultrasound examination of the ovary. Ultrasound scanning of the ovary during this developmental stage will usually visualize the follicle when about 7 mm in diameter, and its normal growth followed with rupture, once the follicle is between 18 and 24 mm in diameter.

Ovulation tends to occur 24–36 hours after the oestradiol peak

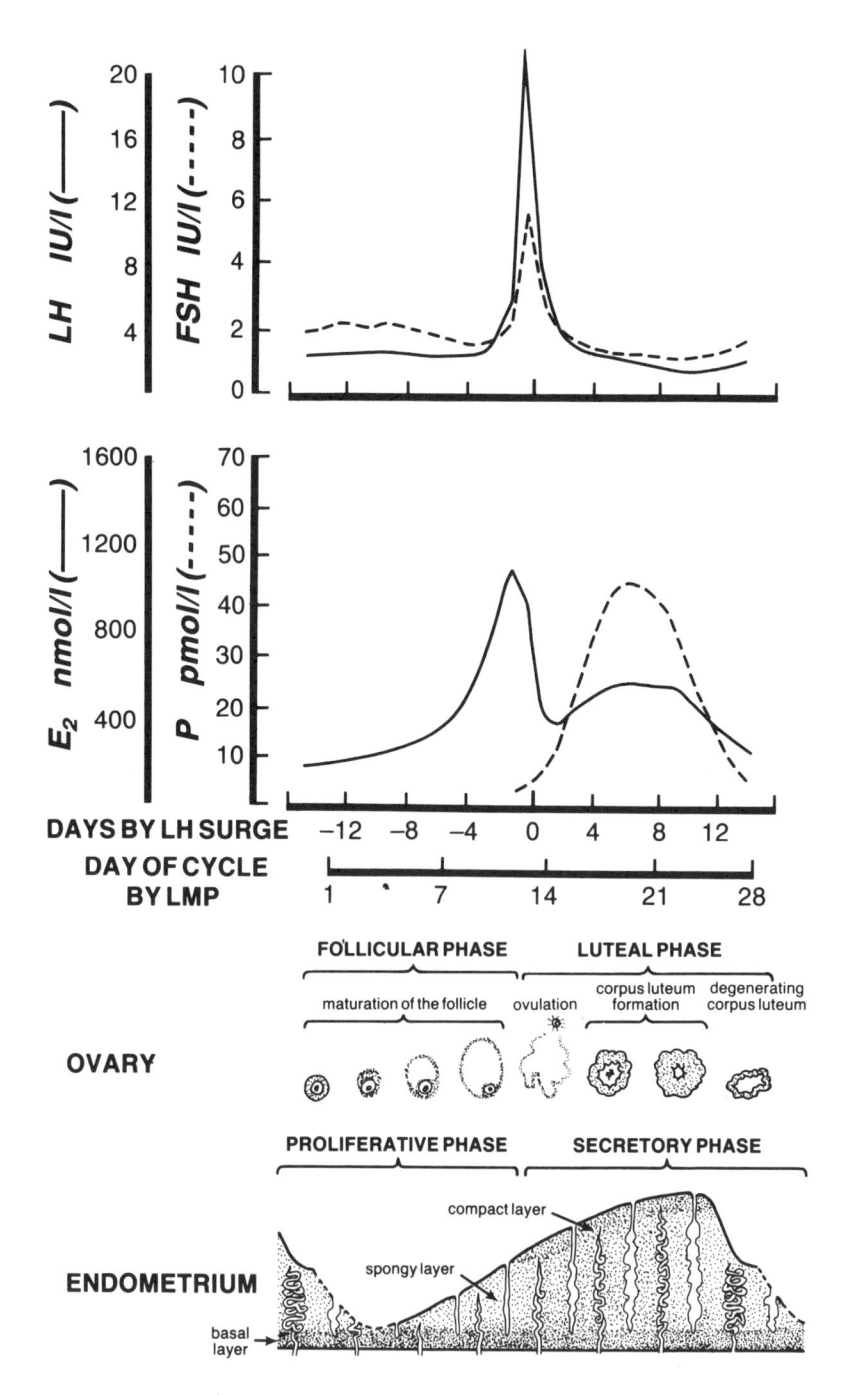

Figure 10.2 Changes during the menstrual cycle.

and 20–22 hours after the LH peak. The presence of a small quantity of progesterone and prostaglandin are necessary for the rupture of the follicle. Inhibition of prostaglandin synthesis at this stage may result in a luteinized unruptured follicle (LUF).

THE CORPUS LUTEUM

The granulosa cells form within the ruptured follicle and the surrounding theca-lutein cells of the ovary form the corpus luteum, which develops a fine network of capillaries and produces large quantities of progesterone under LH stimulation. The main source of progesterone in the luteal phase is the corpus luteum.

The plasma progesterone production appears to reach a peak about 8 days after ovulation, after which the corpus luteum becomes less sensitive to LH and progesterone production falls. Falling progesterone levels result in menstruation. If conception has taken place then the conceptus produces HCG, which further stimulates progesterone production.

CHANGES IN THE ENDOMETRIUM

The menstrual endometrium is thin and dense and has two components, a basal layer, tightly adherent to the myometrium and relatively unchanged throughout the cycle, and a spongy layer, containing blood vessels, glands and stroma.

Early Proliferative Phase

Under oestradiol stimulation the glands in the spongy layer become more prominent, narrow and tubular. The stroma becomes more oedematous and the whole layer tends to form a continuous lining (Figure 10.2).

Late Proliferative Phase

The stroma continues to expand until the endometrium is 3.5–5.00 mm thick (Figure 10.2).

Early Secretory Phase

Progesterone now exerts its influence on the glands which become more tortuous, and the spiral vessels begin to coil and small vacuoles appear (Figure 10.2).

Mid Secretory Phase (Implantation Phase)

The spiral vessels are more tightly coiled and engorged, while the prominent glands are now secreting glycogen. Three layers can be distinguished: the *spongiosum*, the *oedematous stroma*, which is the largest (middle) layer with tightly coiled spiral vessels, and the *superficial* layer. If implantation does not occur then endometrial breakdown takes place (Figure 10.2).

Late Secretory Phase

The levels of prostaglandin F2α rise in the endometrium until at menstruation the ratio of prostaglandin F2α to prostaglandin E2 exceeds 25 to 1. The spiral arteries constrict under the influence of locally produced prostaglandin F2α. The upper part of the spongiosum layer becomes avascular. The interstitial fluid that was causing the oedema is resorbed and small interstitial haemorrhages develop. Eventually these haemorrhages strip off the spongy layer of the endometrium producing menstruation.

Ultrasonography

These changes can be observed by a skilled ultrasonographer with a good machine, who can monitor the thickening of the endometrium and changes in appearance. Early in the proliferative phase the lining is seen as a thin white line and in the late proliferative phase, due to oedematous stroma and the superficial layer, a double layer or ring is produced on ultrasound. In the secretory phase, the endometrium becomes brighter with loss of the darker inner area. Thus, occasionally, a discrepancy is noted between the ovarian and endometrial findings.

Endometrial Proteins

Recent work has shown that these proteins, which have been identified during research into pregnancy, may have a possible role to play in our understanding of other problems, such as infertility, recurrent abortion and, possibly, menorrhagia. Gradually, by using sophisticated biochemical techniques, it has become apparent that the various proteins are the same or very similar. Thus, α_1 PEG/PP12/CAG 1 and PAMG 1 are probably the same and α_2PEG/PEP/AUP/PP14/CAG 2 and PAMG 2 are also synonyms for the same protein. α_1PEG is found in preovulatory follicular fluid and in late luteal phase endometrium, while α_2PEG is the major secretory protein of the mid to late luteal phase.

11

Puberty

INTRODUCTION

In 1755 Dr Samuel Johnson defined puberty as 'the time of life at which the two sexes begin first to be acquainted'.

Definitions:
    Puberty is the beginning of sexual maturity.
    Menarche is the first menstruation.

Menstruation occurs at a relatively late stage in puberty, i.e. one to two years after pubic and axillary hair growth and breast development have started, and after the peak height velocity has occurred. The changes in puberty have been defined and classified by Tanner, stage 1 being the pre-pubertal stage and stage 5 the adult stage. The average times for these changes are shown in Table 11.1.

PHYSICAL SIGNS OF PUBERTY

The Breast

Breast development is usually the first sign of the onset of puberty (Figure 11.1). Initially, at *thelarche*, the breast bud develops, the nipple starts to grow (stage 2), and the breast gradually becomes

Table 11.1 Mean timing of puberty

Development	Stage	Average age (years)
Breasts	2	11
Pubic hair	2	11.5
Breasts	3	12
Pubic hair	3	12
Peak height velocity		12.5
Pubic hair	4	12.75
Menarche		13
Breasts	4	13.5

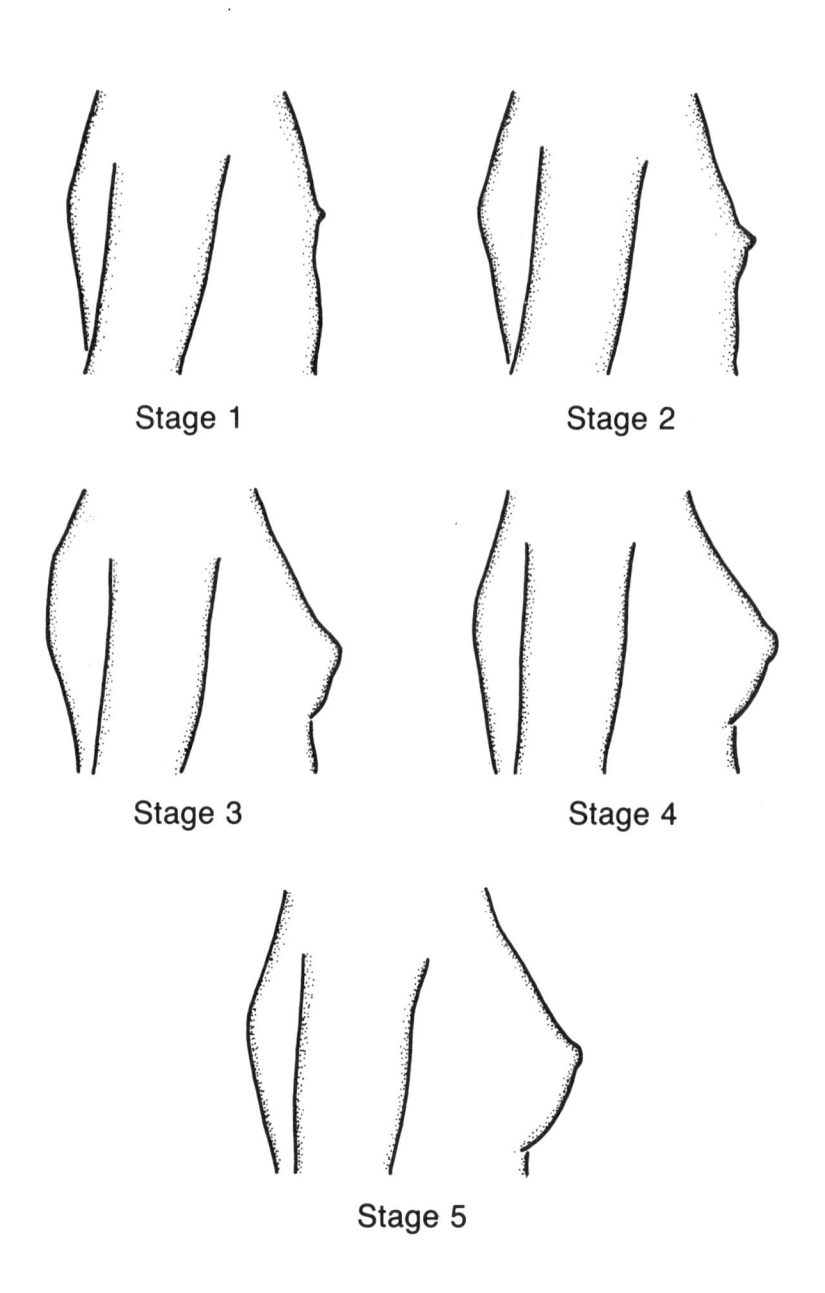

Figure 11.1 Breast development in puberty.

more rounded (stage 3). As the breast size increases the nipple and areolar start to project forward (stage 4) until the full adult form is reached (stage 5). Breast development usually starts between 9 and 13 years and takes about 4 years to become complete.

Pubic Hair

Pubic hair development starts with a few hairs on the mons pubis and vulva (stage 2) which develop into a sparse thin triangle (stage 3), gradually widening out (stage 4) and thickening until the angles are filled out, and the adult distribution is reached (Figure 11.2).

Axillary Hair

Axillary hair develops at the same time as the pubic hair.

Uterus

Changes are also observed in the uterus. At 5 years of age the ratio of the length of the cervix to the body of the uterus is 2:1, but at puberty the body increases in size and in the adult form the ratio is 1:2.

Height

Around the time of puberty, there is also a growth spurt until the adult height is reached when the epiphyses fuse. Usually there is very little further growth in height after regular menstruation is established.

HORMONAL CHANGES

FSH and LH levels are high at birth, after which they fall and levels remain low in childhood, though the level of LH is slightly higher than FSH. The first steroid to increase is *dehydroepiandrosterone (DHA)* which starts to rise between the ages of 6 and 8 years. FSH levels rise before LH. During puberty, there are episodic surges of LH during sleep, which are related to the phases of sleep, and levels are about three times higher than when the child is awake. As these surges can be observed in patients with

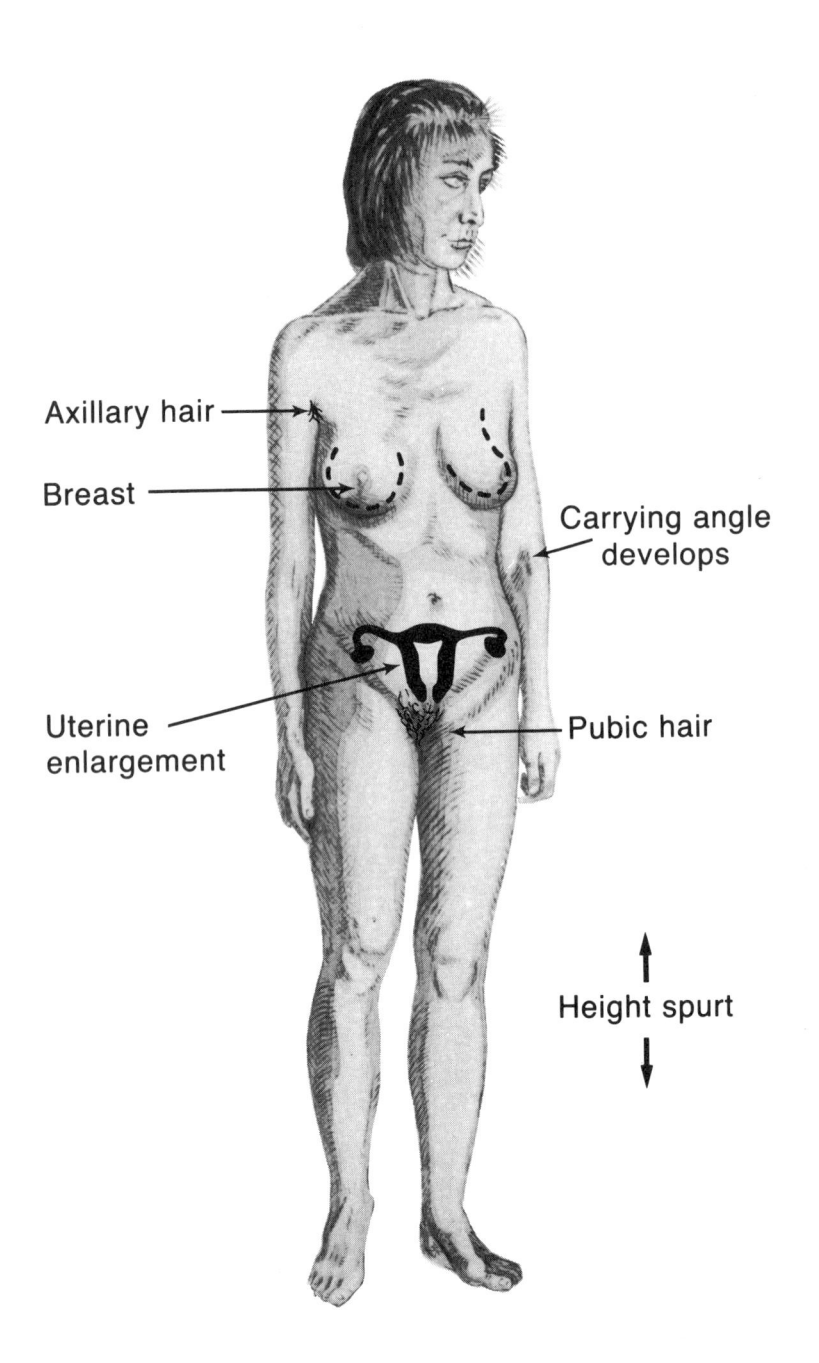

Figure 11.2 Changes at puberty.

gonadal dysfunction the ovaries cannot be the initiator of these changes in gonadotrophins. In the absence of GnRH pulses, there are low FSH and LH levels which serve to stimulate the GnRH pulses. The time comes when oestradiol in particular, but also progesterone, have stimulated enough changes in the endometrium to allow endometrial shedding. These initial cycles are anovulatory and may be heavy, and it usually takes 2 to 3 years for normal menstrual cycles to develop (Table 11.2).

Table 11.2 Hormone levels before menarche

Hormone	Birth	Childhood	6–8 years	10–12 years	Menarche
FSH	High	Low	Rising	Normal	Normal
LH	High	Low	Low	Rising (night surges)	Normal
Oestradiol	—	—	DHA rises	Rising	Normal
Progesterone	—	—	—	Rising	Normal

Ultrasound of the pelvis of a prepubertal child will occasionally reveal a small ovarian cyst, which can be regarded as normal. During puberty the ovary develops numerous small cysts, forming the 'multifollicular' ovary. This is normal in the pubertal girl but abnormal in the adult and suggests that amenorrhoea is related to weight loss.

MENARCHE

The mean age of menarche in the United Kingdom is about 13.2 years. Various factors influence the age of menarche, including social class, race and nutrition. Frische has suggested that there is a critical weight that must be reached for menstruation to occur. In Caucasian girls studied, menarche occurred at 47 kg regardless of height. Menarche will tend to occur earlier in some diseases (Table 11.3).

The first few menstrual cycles tend to be irregular, anovulatory and longer than those in a normal adult.

Table 11.3 Mean ages of menarche depending on disease

Age (years)	Disease
11	Spina bifida
	Congenital abnormalities before 16th intrauterine week (e.g. rubella, thalidomide)
	Epilepsy
12	Physically disabled
	Blind
	Deaf
13	*Normal*
14	Cystic fibrosis
	Mentally retarded
15	Down's syndrome

PRECOCIOUS PUBERTY

Definition
Signs of secondary sexual characteristics showing before the age of 8 years.

Causes

1. Constitutional: genetic, racial and idiopathic. Check for a family history of precocious puberty, with normal hormone profile and no other abnormalities.
2. Neurological: tumours, infections (ask specifically about these), and McCune-Albright syndrome (associated with *café-au-lait* spots and cystic bony changes).
3. Ovarian tumours (high oestrogens and low gonadotrophins).
4. Adrenal tumours (tendency towards hirsutism or even evidence of virilization).
5. Other causes:
   (a) Chorioepithelioma.
   (b) Hypothyroidism: look for cold hands with dry skin.
   (c) Exogenous oestrogen administration.

Investigations

1. Ultrasound of the abdomen to ascertain the state of the ovaries and adrenal glands.
2. Urinary 24-hour oestrogen estimation.
3. X-ray to assess bone age.
4. CAT scan of the brain.

Treatment of Constitutional Precocious Puberty

The aim of treatment is to inhibit hypothalamopituitary activity. Possible treatments are:

1. Progestogens (usually medroxyprogesterone acetate).
2. Anti-androgens (cyproterone acetate).
3. 'Anti-gonadotrophins' (danazol).
4. GnRH agonists (recently brought into use).

The difficulty with hormonal treatment is that it does not necessarily stop the irreversible premature fusion of the epiphyses, resulting in short stature. These patients need very careful support from family, friends and teachers to cope with the psychological strain involved in appearing physically to be adult while still actually a child.

Table 11.4 Causes of precocious puberty and delayed menarche

Precocious puberty (before 8 years)	Delayed menarche (after 16 years)
Constitutional	Outflow obstruction
genetic	(delayed menarche only)
racial	Hypothalamic or pituitary failure
idiopathic	Gonadal dysgenesis
Neurological	Androgen insensitivity
tumours	
infection	
McCune-Albright syndrome	
Ovarian tumours	
Adrenal tumours	Hyperandrogenism
Chorioepithelioma	
Hypothyroidism	
Exogenous oestrogen	

DELAYED MENARCHE

Most girls will have menstruated by the age of 16 years. Failure to menstruate by this age is only significant if:
1. There is no sign of sexual development.
2. Full signs of sexual development have been present for a long time and the patient has not yet menstruated.

Causes

1. *Outflow obstruction.* Imperforate hymen: a blue dome appearance at the vulva will suggest a haematometra. Absent vagina: normally secondary sexual characteristic.
2. *Hypothalamic or pituitary failure.* Normal height with absent secondary sexual characteristics.
3. *Gonadal dysgenesis.* Chromosomal — Turner's Syndrome: short stature, webbed neck, wide carrying angle, absent secondary sexual characteristics, shield shaped chest, widely spaced nipples.
4. *Androgen insensitivity.* Normal height, good breast development, sparse pubic and axillary hair, genetically XY, with normal plasma testosterone level but end organ insensitivity to testosterone.
5. *Androgen excess.* Klinefelter's syndrome: congenital adrenal hyperplasia. Tumours: ovarian or adrenal (signs of masculinization).

These causes are summarized in Table 11.4.

Investigations

Physical examination may suggest the cause, but further investigation to confirm the diagnosis will be needed (Figure 11.3). Investigations include:

1. FSH/LH estimations.
2. GnRH test (to differentiate hypothalamic from pituitary causes).
3. X-rays for bone age.
4. Chromosomal analysis.
5. Possible laparoscopy or ultrasound to assess which organs are present.

Puberty 51

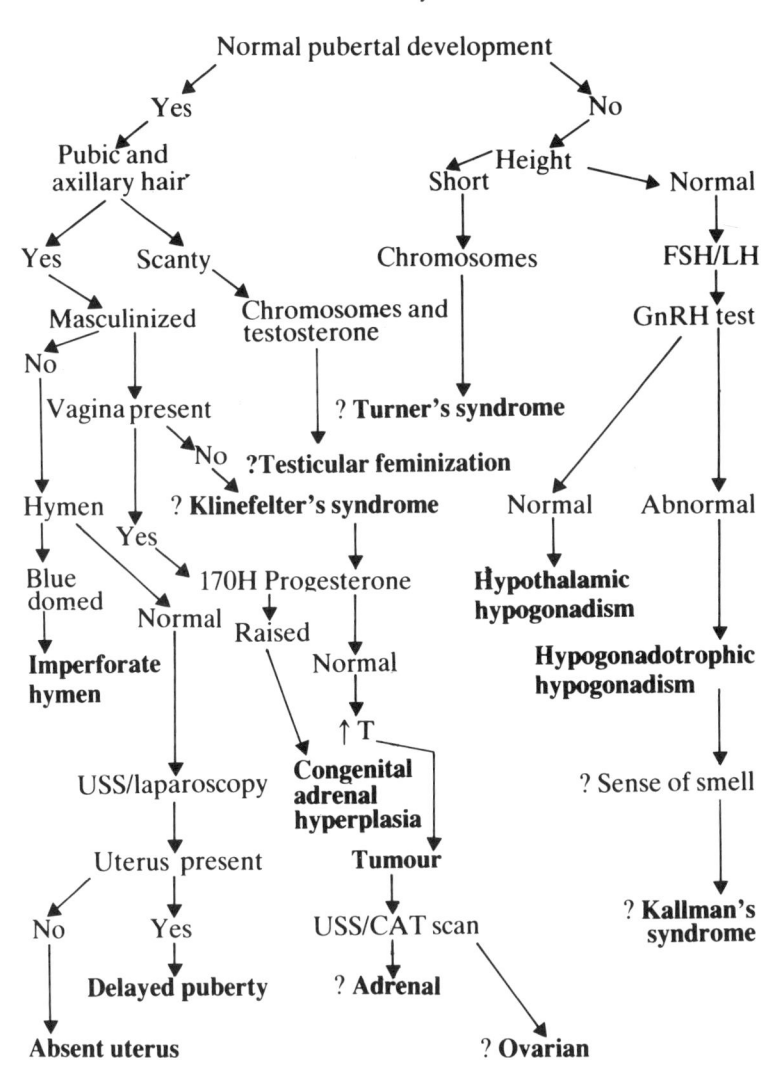

```
                        Normal pubertal development
                   Yes ↙                    ↘ No
        Pubic and                          Height
        axillary hair              Short ↙      ↘ Normal
      Yes ↙     ↘ Scanty           Chromosomes       FSH/LH
    Masculinized    Chromosomes and                  GnRH test
   No ↙              testosterone
   Vagina present        ? Turner's syndrome
                 No ↘ ?Testicular feminization
   Hymen ↓   ? Klinefelter's syndrome    Normal    Abnormal
        Yes ↘
   Blue        170H Progesterone       Hypothalamic
   domed   Normal ↙   ↘ Raised          hypogonadism
                     Normal             Hypogonadotrophic
   Imperforate                          hypogonadism
   hymen              ↑ T
                     Congenital
   USS/laparoscopy   adrenal            ? Sense of smell
                     hyperplasia
   Uterus present    Tumour
   No ↙   ↘ Yes      USS/CAT scan       ? Kallman's
                                         syndrome
       Delayed puberty  ? Adrenal
   Absent uterus               ? Ovarian
```

Figure 11.3   Investigations of delayed menarche.

Treatment

This is dependent on the cause.

1. *Outflow obstruction.* This requires surgical correction.
2. *Hypothalamic or pituitary failure.* Pituitary failure requires gonadotrophin administration. Pulsatile GnRH therapy is proving very effective in hypogonadotrophic hypogonadism. Pulses of 10–20 μg subcutaneously every 90 minutes are used nightly for 8 hours. These patients are best managed in specialized centres.
3. *Gonadal dysgenesis.* Secondary sexual characteristics can be developed, with regular withdrawal bleeds, if cyclical oestrogens are given. Progestogen is added after about a year.
4. *Androgen insensitivity.* Gonadectomy will eventually be required to remove the potential risk of malignant change in the testes.
5. *Androgen excess.* Congenital adrenal hyperplasia requires steroid therapy. Tumours require surgical removal.

12

The Breast

Breast changes occur at puberty, in pregnancy, during lactation and at the menopause.

CHANGES IN SIZE

During puberty the breasts initially develop unequally but once developed they are usually of equal size. During pregnancy the breasts increase in size and occasionally massive hypertrophy is seen. At the menopause the breasts decrease in size. See Figure 12.1.

BREAST CHANGES IN PREGNANCY

The breast undergoes changes during pregnancy. Under the influence of prolactin (from the pituitary) and human placental lactogen (from the placenta), the alveolar cells differentiate into milk secreting cells. However, the high levels of oestrogen and progesterone inhibit significant milk production until after delivery. The initial milk produced is called *colostrum* and full milk secretion usually begins 4–5 days postpartum. Lactation is stimulated by suckling and usually stops as suckling decreases.

GALACTORRHOEA

Galactorrhoea is defined as *inappropriate lactation*.

Common Causes

1. Hyperprolactinaemia.
2. Prolonged nipple stimulation.
3. Oral contraceptives (particularly high dose oestrogen pills).

Hyperprolactinaemia is not always accompanied by galactorrhoea and galactorrhoea is not always accompanied by hyperprolactinaemia.

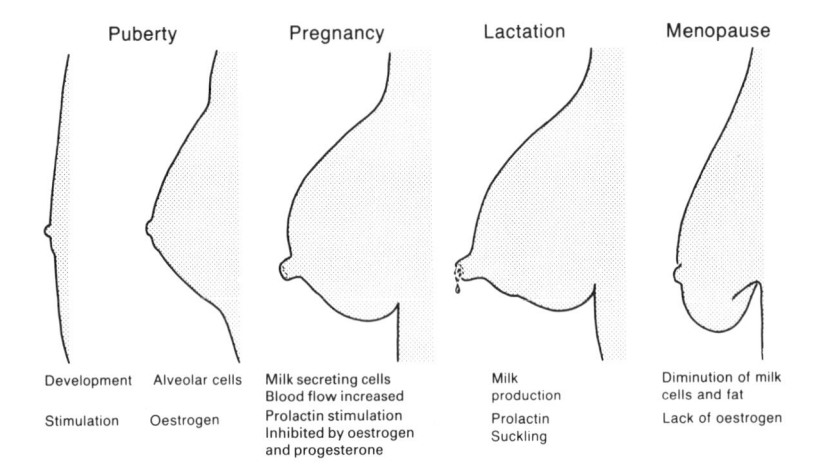

Puberty	Pregnancy	Lactation	Menopause
Development Stimulation	Alveolar cells Oestrogen	Milk secreting cells Blood flow increased Prolactin stimulation Inhibited by oestrogen and progesterone	Milk production Prolactin Suckling	Diminution of milk cells and fat Lack of oestrogen

Figure 12.1 Breast changes.

HYPERPROLACTINAEMIA

The level at which prolactin is considered abnormal will depend upon the population and the assay method used. The normal range for prolactin has a log skew distribution with a long 'tail' in the high range. Older women tend to have higher prolactin levels. In most assessments values over 1000 iu l^{-1} are considered abnormal. These levels will probably not be associated with obvious signs of pituitary tumour until higher levels of 2000 iu l^{-1} or over are reached.

Hyperprolactinaemic amenorrhoea is associated with a hypo-oestrogenic stage, a pale vagina and possible osteoporosis.

Physiological Causes

Pregnancy and lactation.

Pathological Causes

1. Prolactin secreting adenoma.
2. Drugs:
   (a) Phenothiazines
   (b) Tricyclic antidepressants
   (c) Metaclopramide
   (d) Methyldopa.
3. Hypothyroidism.
4. Oestrogen therapy.
5. Acromegaly.
6. Renal failure.
7. Histiocytosis X.

Investigations

1. Thyroid function tests to exclude primary hypothyroidism, as TSH will stimulate prolactin release.
2. X-ray of pituitary fossa to screen for a 'double floor'. If there is any doubt, suggestive of a pituitary tumour, proceed to CAT scan.
3. Visual field testing to exclude tumour encroaching on the optic chiasma.

Treatment

Treatment is with bromocryptine (see page 126). If evidence suggests a tumour, refer to a neurosurgeon.

MASTALGIA

Mastalgia is defined as painful breasts in the absence of significant pathology.

Causes

1. Fibrocystic disease of the breasts.
2. Hypothyroidism.
3. Cyclical changes in the premenstrual syndrome.
4. Neurological—nerve root irritation.
5. Breast carcinoma.

Investigations

1. Examination of the breasts to exclude any masses or cysts.
2. Thyroid function tests.
3. Prolactin estimation.
4. Consider mammogram.

Treatment

1. Danazol 100 mg daily.
2. Bromocriptine may occasionally help.
3. Norethisterone may occasionally help.

13

Amenorrhoea

INTRODUCTION

Definition
Amenorrhoea is either when no menstruation has occurred by the age of 16 years or no menstrual loss has occurred for 6 months.

The former is sometimes referred to as *primary amenorrhoea* and the latter *secondary amenorrhoea*, but these terms may lead to confusion as to the cause of amenorrhoea and are best avoided, especially as 40% of primary amenorrhoea is due to secondary causes.

CAUSES OF AMENORRHOEA

Physiological Causes

1. Prepuberty.
2. Pregnancy.
3. Lactation.
4. Menopause.

All women complaining of amenorrhoea should be presumed pregnant until this has been excluded.

Chromosomal Causes

1. Turner's syndrome (XO) and Mosaics (XO/XX).
2. Testicular feminization (XY) (see page 50).
3. Klinefelter's syndrome (XXY).

Physical Causes

1. Imperforate hymen.
2. Absent vagina.
3. Absent uterus.
4. Absent/streak ovaries.
5. Ashermann's syndrome which is caused by intrauterine adhesions induced by over-enthusiastic currettage.

Serious Systemic Disease

Possibilities are renal failure, tuberculosis or diabetes.

Hormonal Causes

HYPOTHALAMIC

1. Weight loss related amenorrhoea. This occurs when the body weight has fallen to 75% below the ideal, which may mean as little as 10% weight loss in some individuals. Ultrasound of the ovaries will show the classic multifollicular ovaries (MFO) of puberty (Figure 13.2).
2. Anorexia nervosa. The weight loss is accompanied by psychological changes, distortion of body image and food phobias. Ultrasound of the ovaries will show the classic multifollicular ovaries (MFO) of puberty (Figure 13.2).
3. Exercise. This may be related to endorphin release affecting the pulse generator for GnRH. It is more common in runners, rather than swimmers, which suggests that energy expenditure is not the only factor. It occurs with prolonged training.
4. Stress (psychological). This is often short lived in duration, e.g. change in menstrual pattern around school/college examinations.
5. Obesity.
6. Kallmann's syndrome. This is an isolated gonadotrophin deficiency and anosmia, which is more common in males. Patients tend to be tall, have polydactyly, retinitis pigmentosa and cranial nerve palsy.
7. Tumour.

PITUITARY

1. Tumours, particularly prolactin secreting tumours. Hyper-

prolactinaemia is often, but not always, accompanied by galactorrhoea.
2. Acromegaly.
3. Sheehan's syndrome. Avascular necrosis of the pituitary usually caused by prolonged hypotension, i.e. in postpartum haemorrhage.
4. Granulomas.

THYROID

1. Thyrotoxicosis. This causes amenorrhoea with increasing SHBG, resulting in increased oestradiol and an alteration in androstenedione metabolism.
2. Hypothyroidism. This causes amenorrhoea by elevating TSH and hence prolactin, and possibly also by disrupting oestrogen metabolism.

OVARIAN

1. Polycystic ovarian syndrome (PCO).
2. Resistant ovary syndrome. This occurs when there is an insensitivity to FSH/LH, usually due to an autoimmune block of FSH receptors.
3. Premature ovarian failure. When all the potential follicles have developed and undergone atresia before the age of 40.
4. Hormone secreting ovarian tumours.

ADRENAL

1. Congenital adrenal hyperplasia. This is an autosomal recessive disorder of steroid synthesis, which may present at birth with ambiguous genitalia later on or in a milder form with amenorrhoea and hirsutism. The diagnosis is confirmed by a raised 17-hydroxyprogesterone level in the blood. Treatment is with steroids.
2. Tumours.
3. Cushing's syndrome.
4. Addison's disease. This is an antoimmune disease causing adrenal insufficiency, lethargy and pigmentation.

Polycystic Ovarian Syndrome (PCO)

This is the result of a vicious circle of hormonal events. The predisposing factors which start the hormonal circle have not been fully evaluated, but obesity and changes in the ovary may play a role. It is unlikely that there is a hypothalamic or pituitary defect in feedback as these glands respond to oestrogen feedback in the appropriate way, but there may be an abnormality of the pulse generator in the hypothalamus. The prevalence in the normal population of PCOs is unclear.

DIAGNOSIS

Originally, diagnosis depended on the appearance of the smooth white ovaries to the naked eye. Later the finding of a raised LH level and an early follicular LH:FSH ratio that was greater than 3:1 provided a biochemical diagnosis of PCO. With the advent of routine scanning of the ovaries and follicles, it is probable that the ability to assess the ovarian stromal hypertrophy will be used in diagnosis. The woman may be obese and hirsute.

HORMONAL EVENTS: THE VICIOUS CIRCLE

LH secretion stimulates the ovary (particularly the stroma and small sized follicles) to produce androstenedione. This is converted in the body fat to testosterone and oestradiol. The increased testosterone will lower SHBG, which in turn will magnify the increase in oestradiol, resulting in much greater free oestradiol. As the hypothalamopituitary axis is intact, the hypothalamus will respond with an increase in GnRH, resulting in further increases in LH, as the oestrogen priming results in LH release rather than FSH. This increased LH stimulates further androstenedione release to complete the vicious circle (Figure 13.1).

Ultrasound scanning reveals two types of many-cysted ovaries. The classic PCO ovary shows numerous small cysts (2–4 mm) on the outer area and an increased ovarian stroma in contrast to the MFO ovary (Figure 13.2).

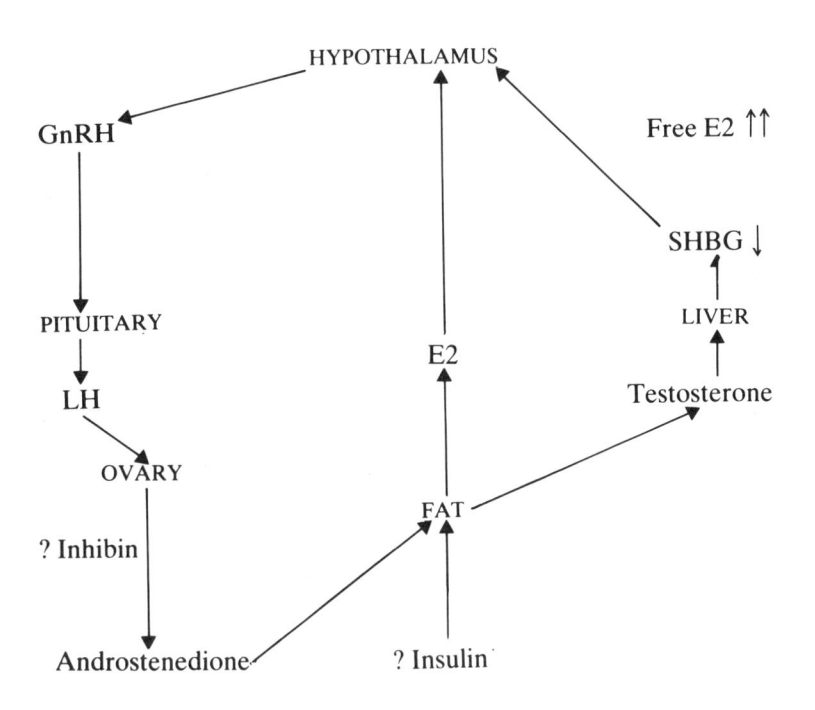

Figure 13.1 The vicious circle of polycystic ovary.

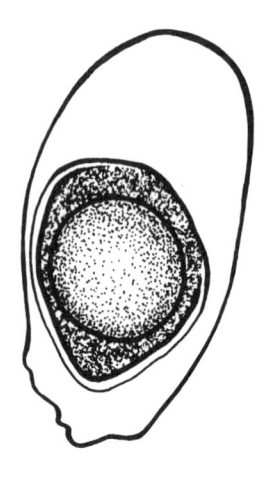

Normal ovary
day 12

Multifollicular ovary
(MFO)
6 or more cysts
4 mm diameter

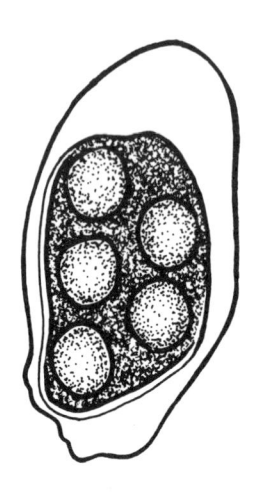

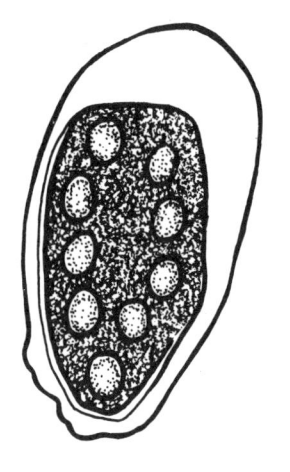

Polycystic ovary
(PCO)
6 or more cysts
2 mm diameter
increased stroma

Figure 13.2 Findings of ovaries on ultrasonic scan.

HISTORY

1. Listen for voice changes: hoarse voice of hypothyroidism, deepening voice in masculinization.
2. Previous menstrual history: particularly previous episodes of amenorrhoea or oligomenorrhoea.
3. Age at menarche/development of secondary sexual characteristics.
4. Hirsutism.
5. Hot flushes or night sweats.
6. Galactorrhoea.
7. Weight loss.
8. Stress.
9. Sense of smell.

EXAMINATION

The signs and symptoms of amenorrhoea are illustrated in Figure 13.3.

INVESTIGATIONS

1. FSH.
2. LH.
3. Thyroid function tests (TFTs).
4. PRL.
5. Ultrasound examination of ovaries.

Possible further tests where appropriate include:

6. Chromosomal analysis.
7. Progestogen challenge test.
8. Testosterone.
9. 17-hydroxyprogesterone.

Figure 13.4 provides an outline of the management of amenorrhoea.

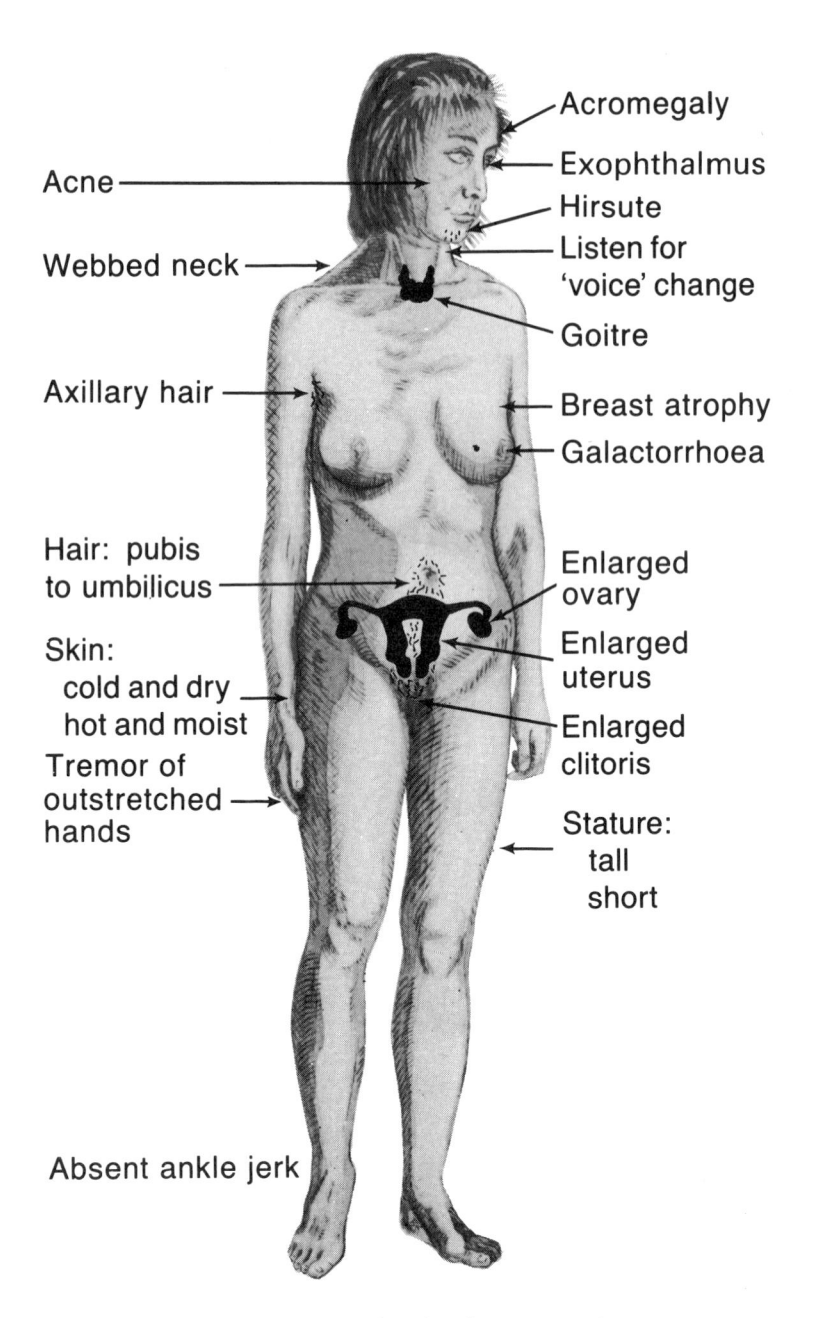

Figure 13.3 Examination for amenorrhoea.

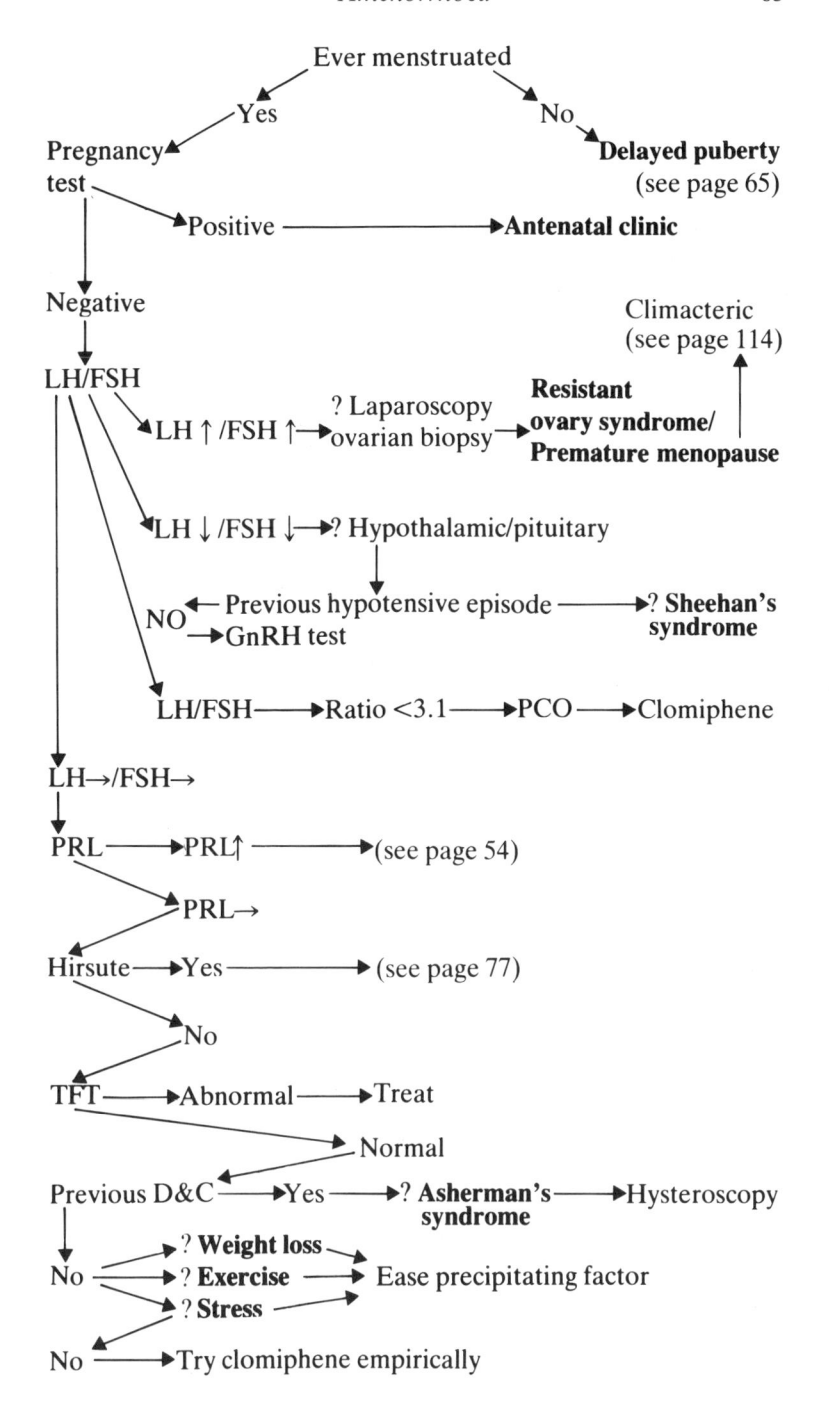

Figure 13.4 The management of amenorrhoea.

TREATMENT

Treatment will depend upon the cause found.

1. *Hypothalamus*. Weight loss and anorexia nervosa: encourage to regain weight. Exercise amenorrhoea: discuss reducing training programme.
2. *Pituitary*. Hyperprolactinaemia: bromocryptine (see page 54). If a tumour is suspected refer to neurosurgeon.
3. *Thyroid*. Thyrotoxicosis: carbimazole or propylthiouracil. Hypothyroidism: thyroxine replacement.
4. *Adrenal*. Cushing's syndrome: metyrapone. Addison's disease and congenital adrenal hyperplasia: steroids. Tumours: refer to a surgeon.
5. *Ovary*. Premature menopausal and resistant ovary syndrome: oestrogen replacement to prevent osteoporosis.

Desensitization of the pituitary with GnRH analogues followed by stimulation of the ovaries with gonadotrophins has been suggested for women anxious to conceive, but it is probably only useful if an IVF pregnancy with donor ova is being considered and luteal support will be required. When there are limited facilities for egg collections for IVF or GIFT, the timing of the cycle needs to be coordinated with the facilities available for egg collection.

PCO is treated with clomiphene (see page 126). If immediate fertility is desired, further methods of ovulation induction may be needed (see page 125) as some women with PCO are very resistant to ovulation induction with clomiphene. Wedge resection of the ovary is no longer used as a method of treatment because, in unskilled hands, it causes adhesions and further impairs fertility.

Clomiphene may help in other cases of hypothalamic amenorrhoea.

POST-PILL AMENORRHOEA

Post-pill amenorrhoea probably does not exist. The amenorrhoea would have developed for whatever reason, if the patient had not been having withdrawal bleeds. Calling the problem 'post-pill amenorrhoea' does not lead to a diagnosis or appropriate treatment.

14

Excessive Menstruation

INTRODUCTION

Definitions
Menorrhagia is excessive menstrual loss.
Metrorrhagia is irregular menstrual loss.
Dysfunctional uterine bleeding is excessive menstrual loss for which no pathological cause can be detected.

Heavy menstruation is a subjective problem. Studies of women complaining of excessive menstrual loss have shown that there is no correlation between the actual blood loss, the number of pads used, haemoglobin levels, nor the state of iron stores when compared with women who consider their menstrual loss to be normal. It is an imprecise and non-objective complaint, although it must not be underestimated as it may be a source of great distress to the patient and her partner.

CAUSES OF MENORRHAGIA

Non-hormonal

1. Carcinoma, endometrial or cervical. This will tend to (but not always) give irregular bleeding.
2. Abnormal surface area. Fibroids and endometrial polyps will increase the surface area of the endometrium.
3. Infection. Pelvic inflammatory disease and endometritis.
4. IUCD. Usage is associated with heavier menstruation which may be due to a local irritant effect and/or to low grade infection.
5. Endometriosis. This may cause increased blood loss particularly in the presence of adenomyosis.

6. Blood dyscrasia.
7. Depression. This brings about stress-related changes in menstruation. The depressed mood will probably also alter the patient's interpretation of her menstrual loss, so that even a normal period seems heavy.
8. Sterilization. This has also been suggested as a cause of increased menstrual blood loss and may represent: a form of 'menstrual intolerance' by the patient once she has decided she wishes to have no more children; the return to 'normal' periods after the lighter withdrawal bleeds of the pill; or a genuine disturbance of blood loss secondary to sterilization.

Figure 14.1 shows the uterine causes of menorrhagia.

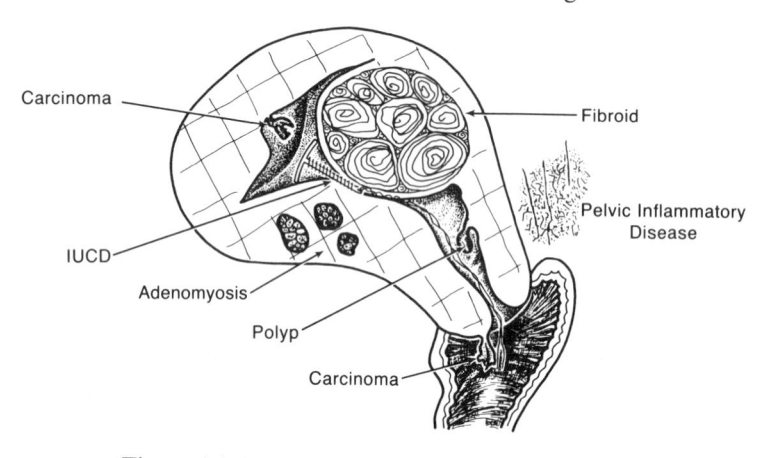

Figure 14.1 Uterine causes of menorrhagia.

Hormonal

1. Polycystic ovaries. Menorrhagia may occur by excessive oestrogenic stimulation of the endometrium (see page 59).
2. Thyroid disease. Both hypothyroidism and hyperthyroidism may be associated with heavy irregular periods.
3. Oestrogen secreting tumours, usually ovarian.
4. Changes in oestrogen and/or progesterone production during the climacteric.
5. Inappropriate prostaglandin production.
6. Administration of hormones.
7. Puberty and climacteric.

HISTORY

1. Duration of the complaint.
2. Regular or irregular menses.
3. Any intermenstrual or postcoital bleeding.
4. Alteration in cycle length.
5. Lengthening of days of bleeding.
6. Contraception used.
7. Recent change in contraception.
8. Cold or heat intolerance.
9. Presence of hot flushes.
10. Recent stress.

EXAMINATION

1. The patient's state when taking the history is important. In particular, is there a suggestion of depression, and any hoarseness in her voice which may suggest hypothyroidism?
2. Signs of anaemia, e.g. pale conjunctiva, skin, lips, tongue.
3. Presence of a goitre.
4. Abdominal mass, e.g. fibroids.
5. Does the cervix appear abnormal, or is there any suggestion of carcinoma of the cervix or a cervical polyp? *Remember* carcinoma of the cervix may be present in young women.
6. Is there an IUCD thread visible?
7. Is the uterus a normal size and shape or is it distorted with fibroids, or fixed retroverted and tender suggestive of endometriosis?
8. Is there any adnexal tenderness?

The signs and symptoms of menorrhagia are illustrated in Figure 14.2.

INVESTIGATIONS

1. A cervical smear should be taken in all women with menstrual irregularity.
2. Endometrial biopsy/currettage should be performed if there is doubt about the possibility of carcinoma of the endometrium,

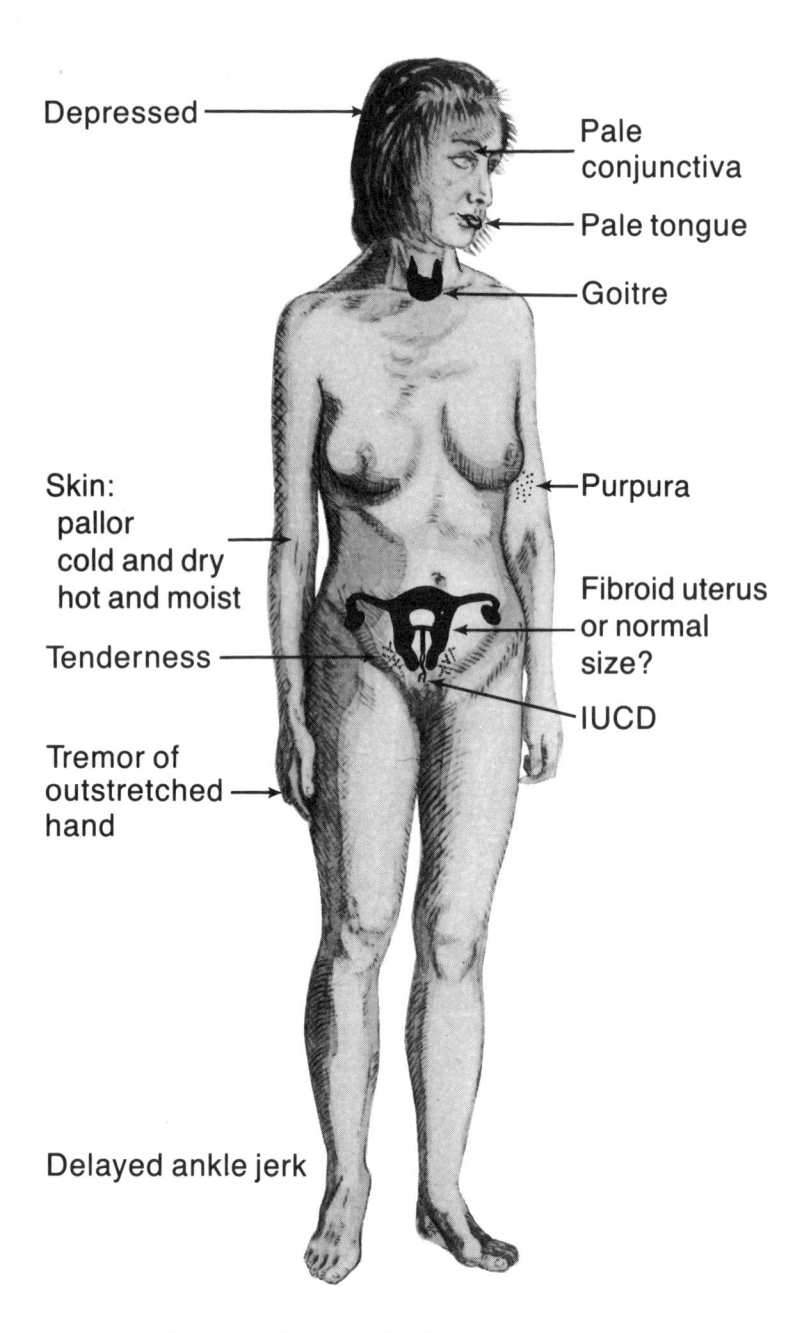

Figure 14.2 Examination for menorrhagia.

particularly in all women over the age of 40 years and those with intermenstrual, postcoital or irregular bleeding.
3. Haemoglobin and blood film.
4. Thyroid function test: if there is any suspicion of thyroid disease, e.g. cold hands, delayed ankle jerks, fine tremor of hands.
5. If a hysteroscope is available it may be used to look for causes of menorrhagia and if the instrument has a suitable attachment, local destruction of the endometrium may be possible.

Dysfunctional Uterine Bleeding

This is diagnosed by exclusion of the other causes. Studies of women with dysfunctional uterine bleeding have failed to show a pathological cause or any consistent abnormal hormonal pattern, the levels of FSH, LH, oestradiol and progesterone being similar to those in normal controls. The role of prostaglandins in the control of menstrual flow is not fully understood, nor have the effects of stress and psychological influences on the perception of menstrual loss been completely evaluated.

Currettage is a diagnostic procedure to exclude serious pathology and not to alter menstrual flow. However, some women need no further treatment either because they have been reassured of no serious pathology, or because the process of currettage can induce changes in the basal layer of the endometrium which alters menstrual flow.

TREATMENT

1. *Progestogens.* By increasing the progestogenic influence on the proliferative endometrium, progestogens may produce a more orderly and synchronized endometrial shedding and reduce blood loss. If the length of the course administered is increased to include the end of the proliferative phase, it may also interfere with oestrogen production, further reducing the menstrual loss, e.g. *norethisterone* or *dydrogesterone* administered from days 19 to 26, or days 10 to 26 depending on the cycle control obtained. *Danazol* is a powerful progestogen, as well as having antigonadotrophin actions, and given in low doses may be effective in menorrhagia.
2. *Prostaglandin synthetase inhibitors.* These also reduce blood

flow and in women anxious to conceive have the advantage that medication is only given during menstruation, e.g. *mefenamic acid*.
3. *Drugs affecting blood clotting*. Fibrinolytic inhibitors, such as *aminocaproic acid*, and systematic haemostatics, such as *ethamsylate*, may be used.
4. *GnRH agonists*. These act by altering GnRH release. They are now being tried in the treatment of menorrhagia, as they have been reported to reduce the size of fibroids, and may prove to offer a real alternative to hysterectomy. However, treatment for longer than 6 months may leave the patient at risk of developing osteoporosis.
5. *Myomectomy*. This can be considered in women who wish to preserve their fertility but have significant fibroids.
6. *Hysterectomy*. This will stop menstrual blood loss, but it is a major procedure and carries serious risks, and should be offered only when medical treatment has failed.

It should be noted that although it is possible to demonstrate significant reduction in blood flow with medical treatment, the patient may still request a hysterectomy to relieve her of recurrent heavy periods. Figure 14.3 summarizes the treatment possibilities.

Excessive Menstruation

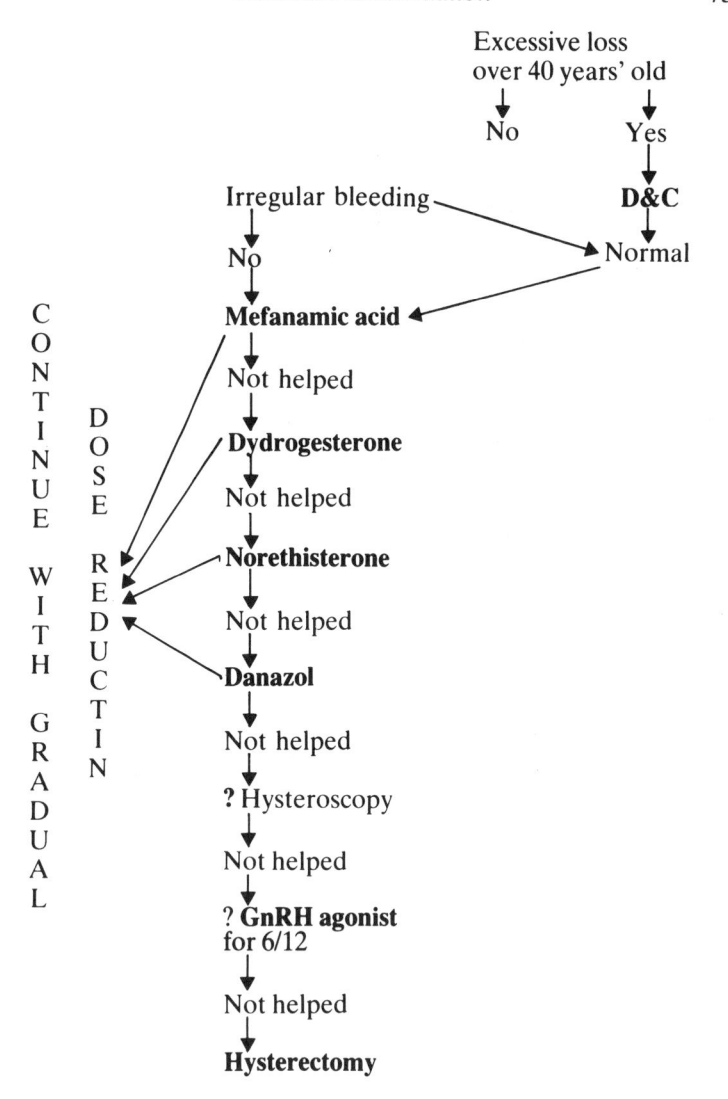

```
                                    Excessive loss
                                    over 40 years' old
                                    ↓            ↓
                                    No           Yes
                                                 ↓
              Irregular bleeding              D&C
                    ↓                            ↓
                    No                        Normal
                    ↓           ←──────────────┘
              Mefanamic acid ←
                    ↓
                Not helped
                    ↓
              Dydrogesterone
                    ↓
                Not helped
                    ↓
              Norethisterone
                    ↓
                Not helped
                    ↓
                 Danazol
                    ↓
                Not helped
                    ↓
              ? Hysteroscopy
                    ↓
                Not helped
                    ↓
              ? GnRH agonist
                for 6/12
                    ↓
                Not helped
                    ↓
              Hysterectomy
```

(CONTINUE WITH GRADUAL DOSE REDUCTION)

Figure 14.3 Treatment of dysfunctional bleeding.

15

Dysmenorrhoea

INTRODUCTION

Definition
   Dysmenorrhoea is pain related to menstruation.

Types of Dysmenorrhoea

Primary: occurring in the early years of menstruation, either spasmodic or congestive.
Secondary: occurring after some years of pain-free menstruation.

PRIMARY DYSMENORRHOEA

Spasmodic Dysmenorrhoea

This only occurs in ovulatory cycles. The pain starts with the onset of the menstrual flow, or shortly before, is most severe on the first day and may last 2 or 3 days. The pain is 'colicky' and occurs in the lower abdomen and may radiate to the back and inner thighs. The teenage girl with spasmodic dysmenorrhoea appears pale and sweaty, and reflex vomiting may occur.

Congestive Dysmenorrhoea

There is lower abdominal pain with heaviness and a bloated feeling in the days preceeding menstruation, but the pain increases with the onset of menstruation. The pain is continuous and may be accompanied by migraine, joint pains, nausea or vomiting.

   Possible hormonal explanations include:
1. High basal intrauterine pressure.

2. More frequent uterine contractions.
3. High $PGF_2\alpha$ in the endometrium.
4. High PG metabolites in the circulation.

These suppositions are supported by the fact that pain relief is achieved with PG synthetase inhibitors (PGSI).

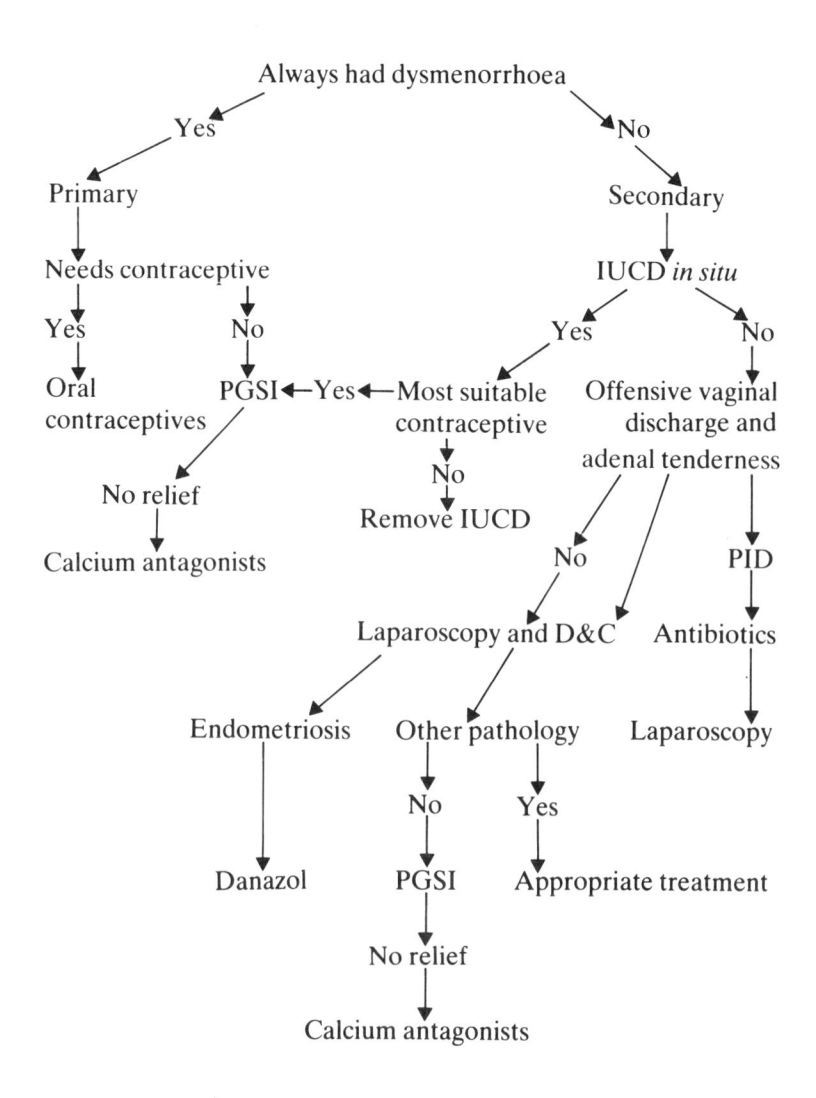

Figure 15.1 The management of dysmenorrhoea.

TREATMENT

1. PGSI, started at the onset of pain.
2. Combined oral contraception.
3. Calcium antagonists may be effective.
4. If no relief is obtained, laparoscopy may be needed to rule out other pathology, especially endometriosis or pelvic inflammatory disease.

There is *no* place for forced dilation of the cervix as a treatment of dysmenorrhoea since this only damages the cervix, leaving the young girl at risk of cervical incompetence in future pregnancies. Figure 15.1 provides a summary of the management of dysmenorrhoea.

CAUSES OF SECONDARY DYSMENORRHOEA

These are outlined in Figure 15.2.

1. Endometriosis.
2. IUCD.
3. Endometrial polyp.
4. Submucous fibroid.
5. Dysfunctional bleeding; the passage of large fragments of endometrium passing through the cervix may cause pain (clot colic).

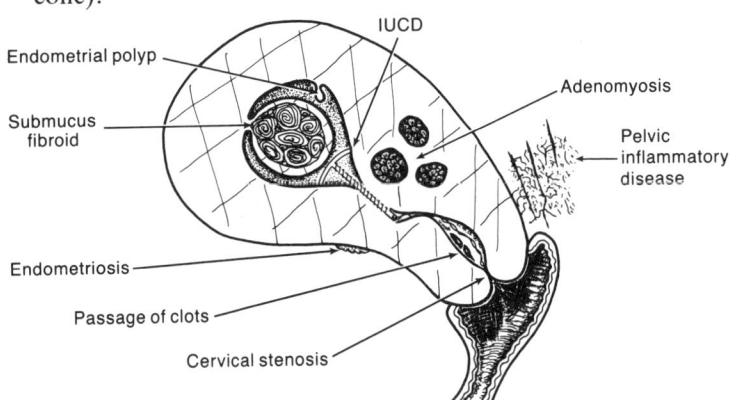

Figure 15.2 Causes of secondary dysmenorrhoea.

TREATMENT

This depends on the cause.

16

Hirsutism

INTRODUCTION

Definition:
Hirsutism is excessive, hormonally controlled hair growth.

There are great differences in both the 'normal' amount of hair and the perception of how much hair is attractive. In Westernized societies the absence of visible hair is considered to be a prerequisite of beauty. The Japanese and Oriental groups have much less facial and body hair than the Mediterranean and Indian races. In anorexia nervosa the body becomes covered in soft light hairs (lanugo), similar to that seen in newborn babies; this must *not* be confused with the abnormal hair growth which is being considered in this chapter.

The Biology of Hair Growth

Each follicle has three phases in a cycle of growth:

1. *Anagen:* the growing phase.
2. *Catagen:* the involuting phase.
3. *Telogen:* the resting phase.

The length of time the hair follicle stays in each phase is variable, hence the time taken to show any response to treatment will be slow. The number of hair follicles per unit area varies between ethnic groups.

Hair growth which is influenced by sex hormones is found on:

1. The face
2. The lower abdomen
3. The anterior thigh
4. The chest
5. The breast
6. The axillae
7. The pubic region.

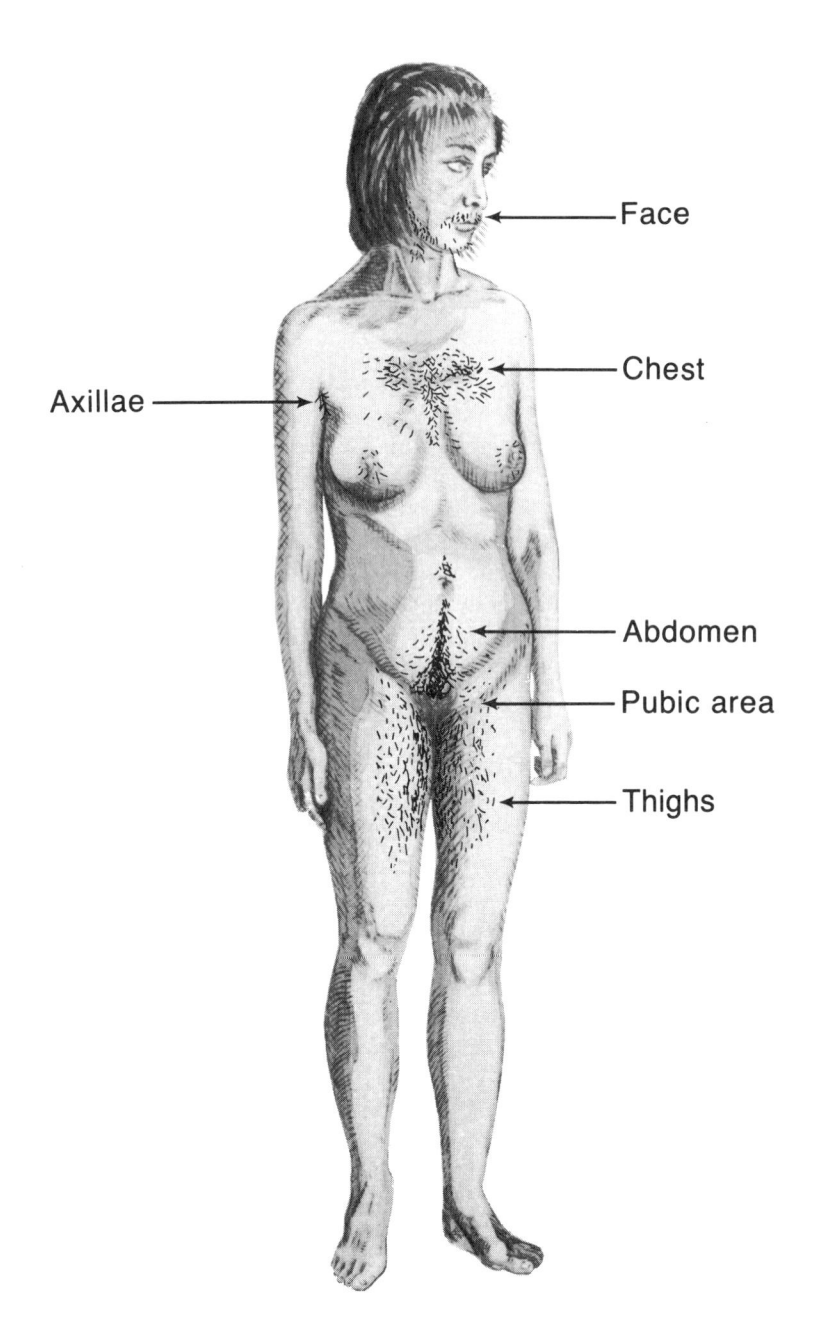

Figure 16.1 Sites of hair under hormonal control.

Figure 16.1 shows the sites of hormonally controlled hair growth. Thus excessive hair on the forearms and calves, without excessive hair in the other areas, is not hormonally controlled, and will respond poorly to hormonal therapy.

Hair growth is influenced by:

1. Androgens (these make the hair thick, dark and curly).
2. Oestrogens (these make the hair finer, straighter and lighter in colour).
3. Pregnancy (this tends to lead to synchrony in telogen and postpartum alopecia).
4. Temperature.
5. Blood flow.
6. Oedema.

CAUSES OF HIRSUTISM

1. *Familial* and *racial*.
2. *Idiopathic*. In this condition there is often a low SHBG and a normal testosterone, thus increasing the free testosterone.
3. *Physiological*. Premenstrually SHBG is low and there may even be a small increase in testosterone secretion.
4. *Iatrogenic*. The administration of androgens as treatment for loss of libido in postmenopausal women. The administration of progestogens, corticosteroids and ACTH may also be implicated.
5. *Pituitary*. Acromegaly. Hyperprolactinaemia.
6. *Thyroid*. Hypothyroidism.
7. *Adrenal*. Androgen secreting tumours:
    Cushing's syndrome. This may be iatrogenic (from excessive administration of steroids) or idiopathic.
    Congenital adrenal hyperplasia (see page 31)
8. *Ovarian*. Polycystic ovary syndrome (see page 59).
    Androgen secreting tumour.

HISTORY

1. Duration of problem.
2. Time of onset.

(a) Since puberty.
(b) Suddenly over a few months (this is suggestive of a tumour).
3. Ethnic background.
4. Drugs taken/creams used (excessive use of steroid creams will result in absorption of steroids).
5. Menstrual upset (this is very common in hirsute women).

EXAMINATION

1. Evaluation of the severity of the problem. The full degree of the problem may not be adequately assessed by casual observation because the patient can successfully camouflage her hirsutism.
2. Distribution of hair over hormone-sensitive areas.
3. Characteristics of the hair:
   (a) Coarse
   (b) Pigmented
   (c) Long
4. Evidence of treatment (scars from badly performed electrolysis, septic spots suggestive of plucked hairs, stubble from shaved hairs, bleached hairs).
5. Receding temporal hairline.
6. Acne.
7. Increased muscle bulk.
8. Clitorimegaly.
9. Breast atrophy.
10. Psychological effect on the patient in relation to the extent of the problem.

Figure 16.2 illustrates the signs and symptoms of hirsutism.

Hirsutism 81

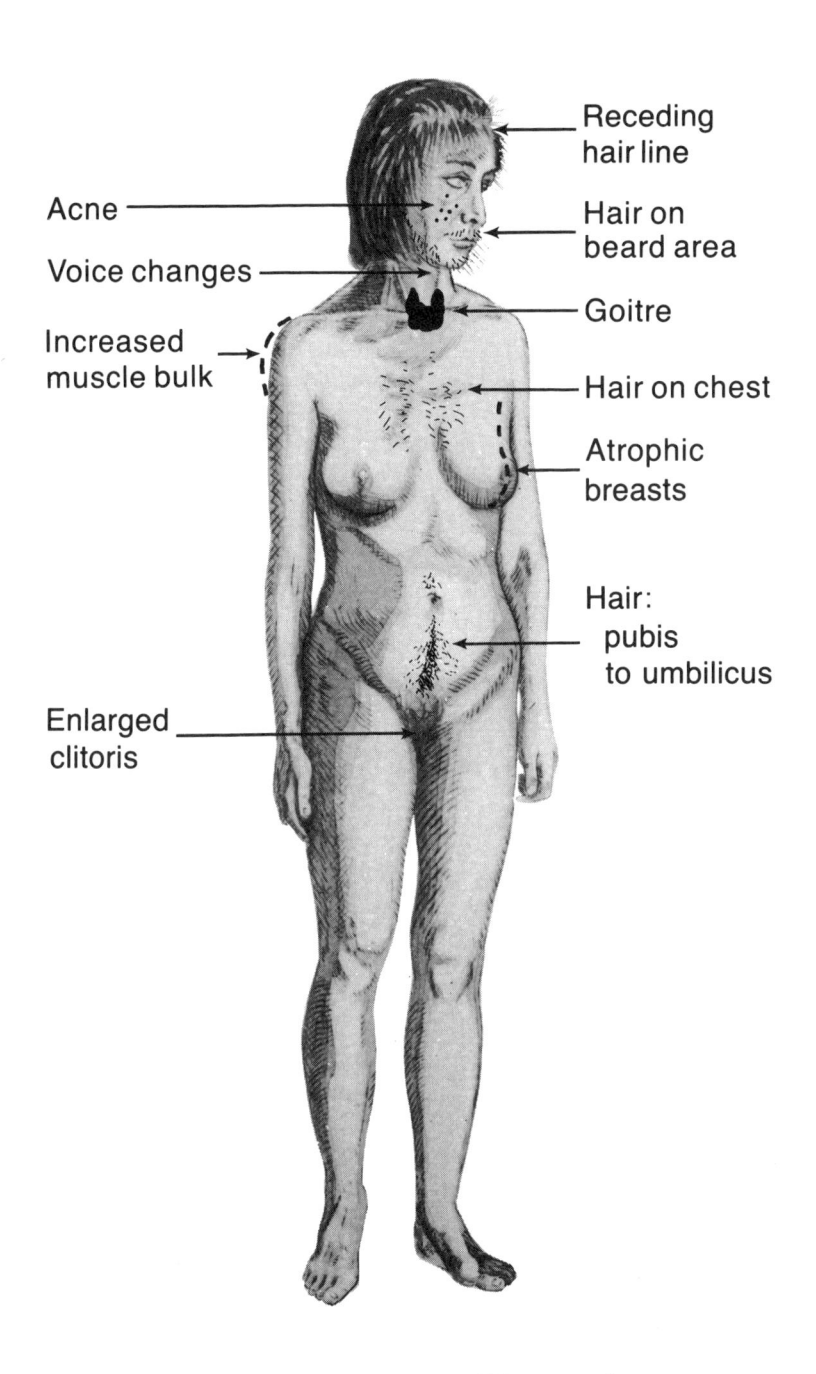

Figure 16.2 Examination of hirsute patient.

INVESTIGATIONS

1. Testosterone
2. SHBG
3. Androstenedione (if available)
4. FSH/LH and ratio
5. PRL
6. Thyroid function tests

If the degree of hirsutism is severe and the cause not obvious, further investigations are required to assess the adrenal glands, e.g. dexamethasone suppression. For a diagnostic summary see Figure 16.3.

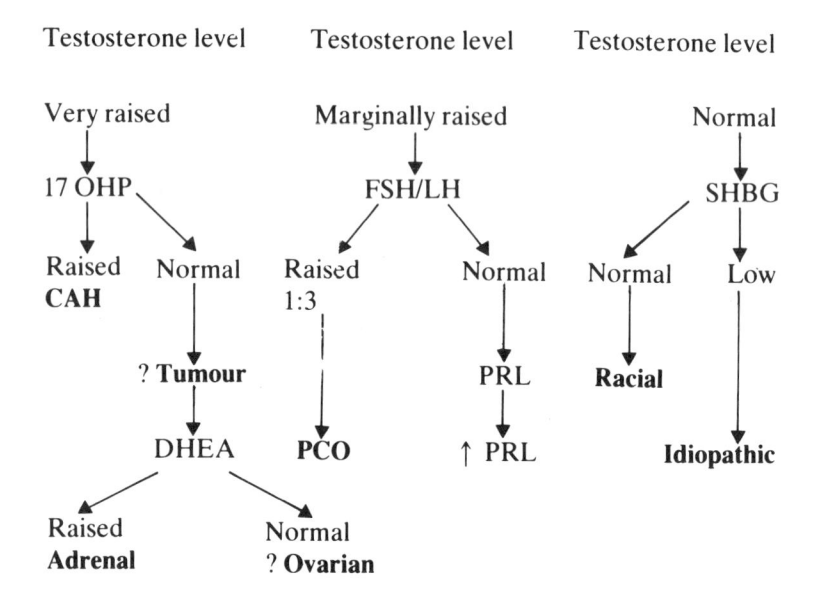

Testosterone level — Very raised → 17 OHP → Raised: **CAH**; Normal → ? **Tumour** → DHEA → Raised: **Adrenal**; Normal: **? Ovarian**

Testosterone level — Marginally raised → FSH/LH → Raised 1:3 → **PCO**; Normal → PRL → ↑ PRL

Testosterone level — Normal → SHBG → Normal: **Racial**; Low: **Idiopathic**

Figure 16.3 Diagnosis of hirsutism.

TREATMENT

If testosterone and androstenedione levels are very high the cause must be presumed to be due to a tumour, which must be found and removed. In the other cases the cause, if found, should be treated in the usual way.

Idiopathic Hirsutism

This is treated with cyproterone acetate and ethinyl oestradiol. Cyproterone acetate is an antiandrogen and potent progestogen, which will cause feminization of a male fetus and therefore should not be taken during pregnancy, or if a possibility of pregnancy exists. The addition of ethinyl oestradiol not only helps to make the regimen contraceptive, but it also stimulates SHBG production and therefore reduces the free testosterone. It also affects the hair follicle by a direct action.

The usual regimen is:

Cyproterone acetate 50 mg days 5–15
Ethinyl oestradiol 50 mg days 5–25

A preparation of cyproterone acetate at a much lower dose is available in the form of the contraceptive pill 'Diane'. It does not seem to be as effective for the severe sufferer but should be considered for the mildly hirsute, acne suffering teenager who needs contraception.

The psychological management of the patient is important; helping them to overcome their embarrassment is an essential element of successful treatment. Occasionally the use of polaroid photographs before and after treatment can help, because patients often cannot remember how bad they were before treatment as the changes occur only slowly.

1. Low dose dexamethasone is not so effective and has the usual side-effects of steroids. However, the Committee of Safety on Medicines does *not* recommend the prolonged use of spironolactone, which may be carcinogenic.
2. Cimetidine and spironolactone are being assessed as treatments, and may be useful.
3. High dose oestrogen oral contraceptive pill.

Non-hormonal Methods

1. Camouflage creams
2. Bleaching
3. Shaving
4. Waxing
5. Electrolysis.

17

The Premenstrual Syndrome

INTRODUCTION

Definition
Regularly recurring symptoms in the same phase of the menstrual cycle (premenstruum) with a symptom-free phase in the postmenstruum.

A premenstrual exacerbation of an underlying disease is therefore not, by definition, premenstrual syndrome (PMS) but is sometimes referred to as *menstrual distress*, as the patient will have symptoms *throughout* the menstrual cycle.

DIAGNOSIS

The definition of PMS depends not upon the type of symptoms but on the *timing of symptoms*.

Thus the diagnosis relies entirely on confirming the *timing* of the symptoms and the phase of the menstrual cycle, and verifying the symptom-free postmenstrual phase. This is best done by making the patient prospectively chart her symptoms and her menstruation for about 3 months prior to commencing treatment. A past history of postnatal depression, immediately prior to the onset of PMS, may be significant. There appears to be a recovery stage in postnatal depression (PND) when the patient is only depressed premenstrually. Usually she will go on to recover completely.

In PMS there must be a symptom-free period in the postmenstruum. Some women will be 'higher' complainers than others but could still have genuine PMS. The diagnosis will then depend both on the timing of the symptoms and the increase in the symptoms. A 'high' complainer with only a small rise in symptoms premenstrually probably does not have PMS but a large increase in symptoms would suggest genuine PMS. The patients are both difficult to differentiate and to treat.

PREVALENCE

Studies by sociologists have found that most women claim to have some symptoms premenstrually. However, it has been found that only 20–25% of women referred to PMS Clinics have the diagnosis confirmed by charting their symptoms. The diagnosis must always be made *prior* to starting treatment.

SYMPTOMS

Over 150 symptoms have been recorded. It is the *timing* of the symptoms and not the type that is important. The most common symptoms are summarized in Figure 17.1.

Psychological

1. Depression. This can sometimes lead to attempted suicide.
2. Irritability. This can be very variable in severity but it can result in baby battering and aggressive outbursts.
3. Anxiety. This can produce panic attacks.
4. Lethargy.
5. Breast tenderness.

Dermatological

1. Acne.
2. Boils.
3. Urticaria.

Gastrointestinal

1. Abdominal bloating.
2. Sugar cravings.
3. Alcoholic bouts.

Neurological

1. Headache.

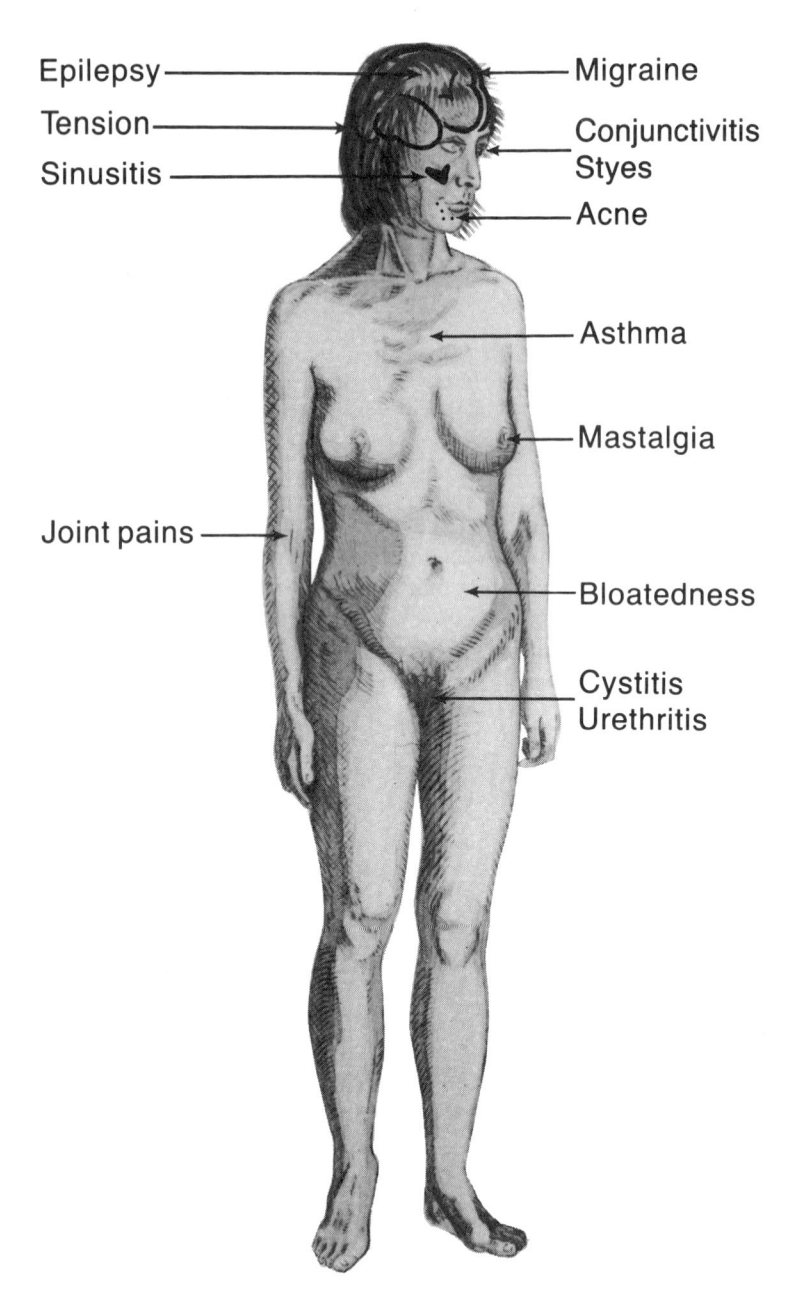

Figure 17.1 Symptoms of premenstrual syndrome.

2. Classical migraine.
3. Epilepsy.

Orthopaedic

1. Backache.
2. Joint pains.

Ophthalmological

1. Conjunctivitis.
2. Styes.

Otorhinolaryngological

1. Sinusitis.
2. Hoarse voice.

Respiratory

1. Asthma.

Urological

1. Cystitis.
2. Urethritis.

CAUSES

These are unknown, although many different hypotheses have been put forward. There are several suggested explanations.

Progesterone Deficiency

This theory is based on the fact that the symptoms occur at the time of luteal progesterone secretion. Convincing proof of this theory is lacking, although the fault may lie with the progesterone receptors.

Vitamin and Mineral Deficiencies

Vitamin B6 (pyridoxine), magnesium and zinc deficiencies have all been suggested as causes of PMS; however it does seem unlikely that any dietary deficiency is present only at some days in the menstrual cycle and not others.

Hyperprolactinaemia

As prolactin is a stress hormone it will tend to be increased in women who are very upset at the time of testing.

Endorphin Disturbance

This has been suggested but not proven.

Prostaglandin Disturbance

This has also been suggested; both a deficiency and an excess have been hypothesized.

TREATMENT

The first consideration is whether treatment is necessary or warranted. Mild personality changes premenstrually may be very common and may not justify the complications of treatment. Once the symptoms have reached the stage of disrupting the lives of the patient and her family, treatment is justified. Figure 17.2 summarizes the treatment of PMS.

Mild Symptoms

A clear explanation of the nature of symptoms and their cause may help the patient to understand the problem. Adjustment of lifestyle may be all that is necessary in the premenstruum, for example avoidance of undue stress and plenty of rest.

Small frequent meals, i.e. some complex carbohydrate eaten every 3 hours, is often helpful and may be all that is required.

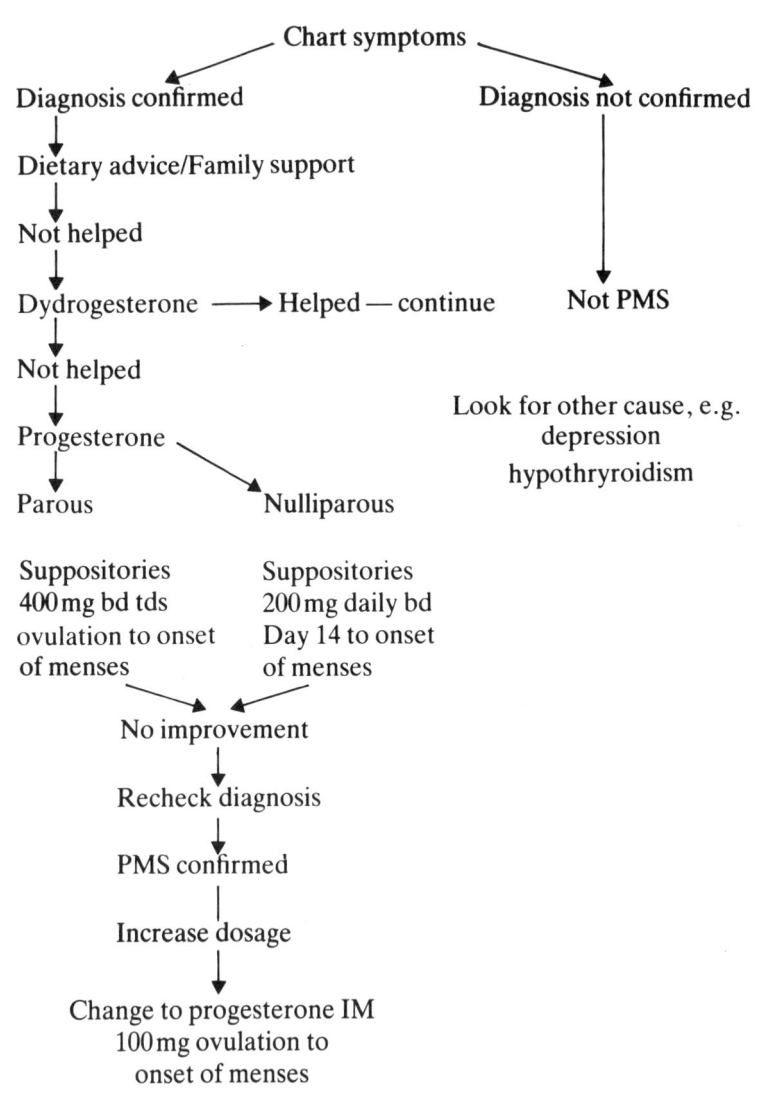

```
                          Chart symptoms
                         ╱              ╲
         Diagnosis confirmed          Diagnosis not confirmed
                 ↓                              ↓
         Dietary advice/Family support
                 ↓                           Not PMS
         Not helped
                 ↓
         Dydrogesterone ──→ Helped — continue
                 ↓
         Not helped                  Look for other cause, e.g.
                 ↓                          depression
         Progesterone ╲                  hypothryroidism
                 ↓       ╲
         Parous          Nulliparous

         Suppositories   Suppositories
         400 mg bd tds   200 mg daily bd
         ovulation to onset  Day 14 to onset
         of menses       of menses
                 ↘       ↙
             No improvement
                    ↓
             Recheck diagnosis
                    ↓
             PMS confirmed
                    ↓
             Increase dosage
                    ↓
         Change to progesterone IM
            100 mg ovulation to
               onset of menses
```

Figure 17.2 Treatment of PMS.

Moderate Symptoms

There are many suggested treatments which reflect the various views held on the causes of PMS.

Progesterone suppositories or injections have been recommended. *Dydrogesterone,* which is an orally active progestogen, is also used.

Vitamin B6 is effective in treating women who suffer depression when taking the pill and therefore has been suggested, but signs of overdosage (lethargy, depression and tiredness) may be similar to the presenting symptoms, and care must be taken to check for the development of peripheral neuropathy.
Oil of Evening Primrose has been advocated for various mild types of depression including PMS.
Prostaglandin synthetase inhibitors are effective for dysmenorrhoea and have also been tried for headaches and joint pains.
Danazol has also recently been reported to help some patients with PMS.

Spironolactone has also been suggested as a treatment for PMS. However the Committee on Safety of Medicines has advised that its use is restricted because of reports of potential carcinogenicity.

LEGAL IMPLICATIONS

The presence of severe PMS may be a mitigating factor in relevant criminal cases in England, but it is not an excuse for committing an illegal act. It is essential to *chart the symptoms* of any patient who complains of PMS and record this in the patient's notes as accurately as possible to refute or confirm the diagnosis before the patient tries to use PMS as mitigation in a court case. PMS must not become a universal mitigating factor in abnegating responsibility in criminal matters. However, there is little doubt that a few patients will have very severe PMS symptoms which may impair their criminal responsibility.

In other countries the question of whether PMS is a legal defence is variable. At the time of writing, no case appears to have been successfully defended in America, for instance, on the basis of a criminal charge.

18

Infertility

INTRODUCTION

Definitions
   Infertility is the failure to conceive after 1 year of unprotected intercourse.
Primary infertility is never having conceived.
Secondary infertility is difficulty in conceiving again, having already conceived on at least one occasion.

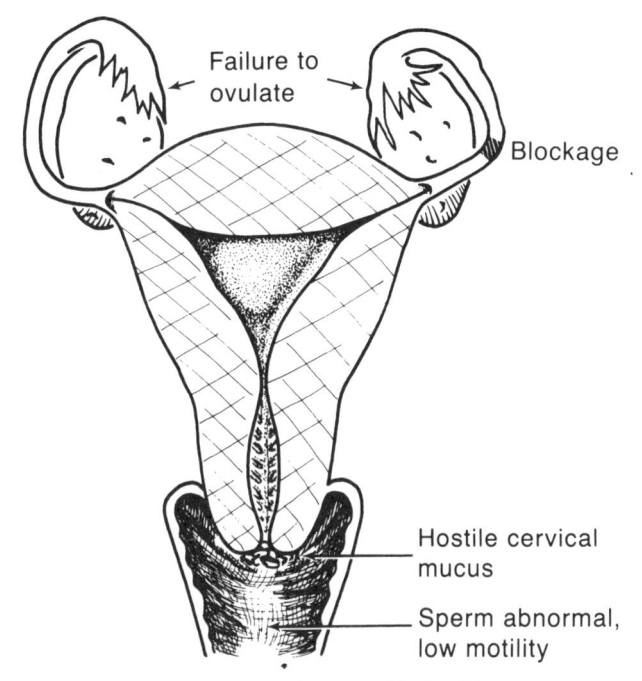

Figure 18.1   Causes of infertility.

The difficulty may lie with the male partner, the female or both, although sometimes no cause can be found with our present methods of investigation and management (see Figure 18.1).

Factors required for conception:
1. Sperm production
2. Ovulation
3. Sperm and ovum to meet successfully
4. Implantation of conceptus.

SPERM PRODUCTION

Sperm Analysis

The sample should be examined within 2 hours and to be satisfactory should have:

1. Volume 2–6 ml
2. Density $40 \times 10^6 - 100 \times 10^6$ sperms ml^{-1}
3. Motility >60% within 2 hours
4. Morphology >60% normal sperm.

Azoospermia is absence of sperm on analysis and may be due to:

1. Blockage of the vas, in which case FSH and LH will be normal.
2. A pituitary gonadotrophin deficiency (usually absent FSH).
3. An abnormality of spermatogenesis in which a raised FSH is usually due to lack of inhibin.

Oligospermia is a low sperm count, which should be repeated at least twice after 2 days' abstinence. The causes of oligospermia are more difficult to assess and treat and should be referred to a specialist in male infertility.

FAILURE OF SPERM AND OVUM TO MEET

This may be due to:

1. Intercourse not occurring.
2. Premature ejaculation.
3. Hostile cervical mucus.

4. Tubal blockage due to infection.
5. Endometriosis.
6. Ovary bound down with adhesions.

Factors 1–3 may be checked by a postcoital test (PCT) (taking a sample from the cervix after having had intercourse the previous night).

Factors 4, 5 and 6 can be checked at laparoscopy by attempting to pass dye through the tubes or by an x-ray of the tubes (hysterosalpingogram: HSG).

ANOVULATION

Ovulation may be detected by daily ultrasound scanning of the ovarian follicle. Demonstrating that it develops and then collapses is positive evidence of ovulation and is the most accurate method available at present.

Ovulation occurs 22–26 hours after the LH peak. Methods of detecting the LH peak by plasma or ultrasensitive urine tests (which are commercially available) will indicate that ovulation is about to occur.

Ovulation may also be inferred by elevated progesterone as demonstrated by a mid-luteal phase blood sample to measure progesterone. Values over 30 nmol l^{-1} 7 days after ovulation is highly suggestive of ovulation with good corpus luteal function.

A basal body temperature (BBT) may be taken each morning before getting up. At ovulation the temperature falls, then rises and remains elevated for some days. This is the least accurate method of assessing ovulation but the simplest and cheapest. It needs a good chart to give a positive result.

The cervical mucus can be checked each day to observe when it becomes thinner and stretchy. This implies ovulation.

Causes

HYPOTHALAMIC

1. Those women with weight loss related amenorrhoea (see page 58).
2. Anorexia nervosa (see page 58).

PITUITARY

3. Hyperprolactinaemia (see page 54).
4. Simmonds'/Sheehan's syndrome (rare) (see page 59).

THYROID

5. Hypothyroidism (see page 59).
6. Hyperthyroidism (see page 59).

ADRENAL

7. Congenital adrenal hyperplasia (see page 59).
8. Cushing's syndrome (adrenal causes are rare).
9. Addison's syndrome (see page 59).
10. Adrenal tumour.

OVARY

11. Resistant ovary syndrome/premature ovarian failure (see page 59).
12. Polycystic ovary syndrome (see page 59). This is also associated with a high abortion rate so that pregnancy rates in treatments with PCO must be assessed as number of live births.
13. Iatrogenic. Taking the oral contraceptive pill.
14. Luteinized unruptured follicle syndrome (LUFS). This can best be diagnosed by ultrasound imaging. For some reason the follicle can be seen to develop normally but it is never seen to collapse, although luteinization takes place as judged by a rise in plasma progesterone.

History

Ideally both partners should be present at the first interview and both should be examined. If the male partner is not present his past medical history, past history of exposure to sexually transmitted disease and any previous children he may have fathered should be ascertained. The fact that the male partner has previously fathered children does not rule out a male factor in the problem, but does make it less likely.

Infertility

A menstrual history is important as amenorrhoea or oligomenorrhoea will accompany many causes of anovulation. N.B. regular menstrual cycles may be anovulatory.

A carefully recorded history of drugs ingested by both partners is important. The possible factors are summarized in Table 18.1.

Table 18.1 History of infertile patient

Male	Female
Past medical	Past medical
Sexually transmitted disease	Sexually transmitted disease
Drugs used	Drugs used
Children fathered	Menstrual
Ejaculation	Gynaecological
	Obstetric

Examination

1. Weight and height
2. Check for signs of hirsutism
3. Check thyroid function
4. Check for signs of galactorrhoea
5. Vaginal examination.

Investigations

1. Seminal analysis/PCT.
2. Assess tubal function by hysterosalpingogram or dye laparoscopy.
3. If the woman is menstruating, perform a mid-luteal progesterone estimation, approximately 7 days before the next menstruation (this is day 21 of a 28-day cycle).
4. If the woman is amenorrhoeic exclude the possibility that she has already conceived, and then investigate (see page 65).
5. Rubella immunity should be checked so as to avoid the awful tragedy of a woman conceiving and then developing rubella, leading to a traumatic chain of events for both the patient and her partner.

Figure 18.2 summarizes the management of infertility.

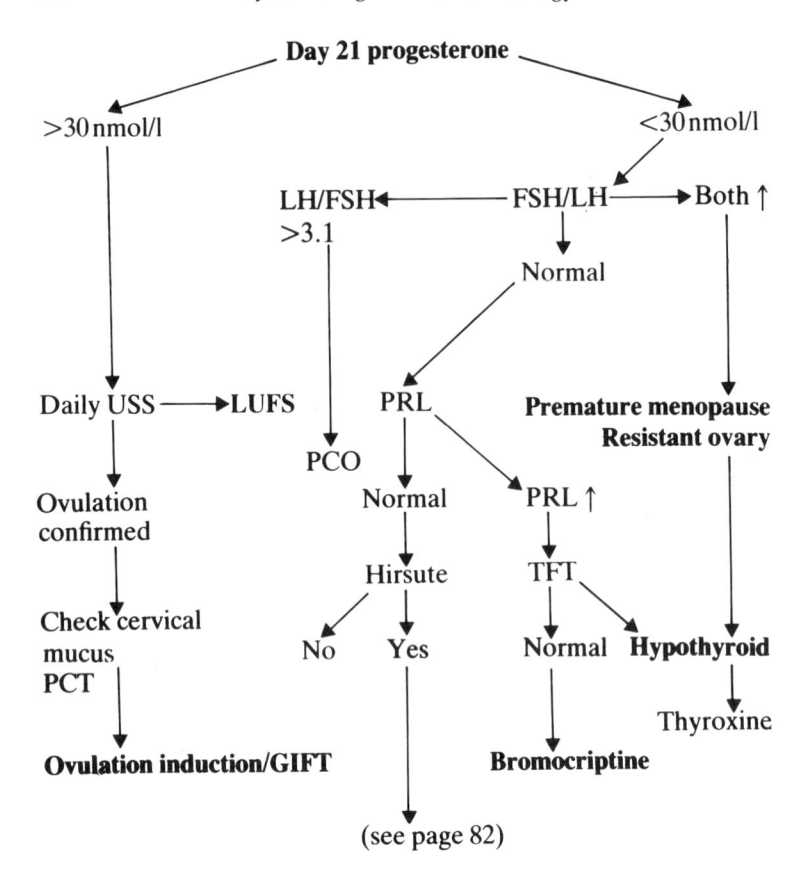

```
                        Day 21 progesterone
          >30 nmol/l                        <30 nmol/l

                    LH/FSH ← FSH/LH → Both ↑
                    >3.1      ↓
                              Normal
                              ↓
   Daily USS → LUFS    PRL        Premature menopause
     ↓                              Resistant ovary
                      PCO
   Ovulation           ↓       PRL ↑
   confirmed         Normal      ↓
     ↓                 ↓         TFT
   Check cervical   Hirsute      ↓
   mucus          No    Yes   Normal   Hypothyroid
   PCT                                    ↓
     ↓                                  Thyroxine
   Ovulation induction/GIFT  Bromocriptine

                    (see page 82)
```

Figure 18.2   The management of infertility.

If the infertile woman is amenorrhoeic she may be given a progesterone challenge test (see page 34) and be asked to take clomiphene 50 mg for 5 days. If she bleeds, ovulation may be checked by a progesterone estimation 14 days after finishing her course of clomiphene.

Treatment

If a clear cause for anovulation is found, this should be treated appropriately. If no adequate explanation can be found, ovulation may be induced by the use of anti-oestrogens, gonadotrophin simulation or GnRH pump.

ANTI-OESTROGENS

By binding to the oestrogen receptors of the hypothalamus and the pituitary, these anti-oestrogen drugs will induce further FSH release to stimulate the developing follicle.

1. Clomiphene 50 mg days 2–6, increasing if necessary to 200 mg.
2. Tamoxifen 10 mg bd days 2–6, increasing if necessary to 40 mg bd.
3. Cyclofenil 200 mg bd days 3–12.

A check of ovulation (usually by serum progesterone estimation) should be made.

GONADOTROPHIN STIMULATION THERAPY

This should only be tried if anti-oestrogen therapy has failed. The dose must be carefully monitored because hyperstimulation can be dangerous: it can result in death, due to the massive shift of fluids from the intravascular space to the ovaries and abdomen, and it carries a high risk of producing multiple pregnancies. Gonadotrophins are administered and follicular growth checked by ultrasound and/or rising urinary or plasma oestrogens. When the follicle has developed, an injection of HCG or LH is given to induce ovulation.

GnRH PUMP

A portable pump allows a syringe to administer pulsed GnRH for a few days in the mid-cycle to increase FSH and LH release. This is most suitable for hypogonadotrophic hypogonadism.

OVULATION INDUCED FOR IN VITRO FERTILIZATION

Many centres undertaking *in vitro* fertilization (IVF), gamete intrafallopian transfer (GIFT) and other related techniques, aim to develop more than one follicle so that they can harvest a number of ova at one time and increase the chance of success. Various regimes are being used for this purpose including 'turning off' (desensitizing) the hypothalamus with GnRH agonists and then administering Pergonal and HCG. Other centres just use

Pergonal alone or clomiphene with an intact hypothalamus, but with slightly differently timed regimes to induce multiple follicles, i.e. the opposite aim from standard ovulation induction therapy where only one follicle is wanted.

IVF involves taking the oocytes (either from the patient herself or a donor) and incubating them with washed sperm and replacing the resultant embryos. GIFT involves replacing the oocytes and washed sperm down the fallopian tube under laparoscopic control.

BROMOCRIPTINE

This is useful only in hyperprolactinaemic anovulation. Once the prolactin has returned to normal, the chance of conception equals that of the normal population. Lisuride is undergoing investigation as an alternative treatment for hyperprolactinaemic women unable to tolerate bromocriptine.

RECURRENT ABORTION

Definition
Recurrent abortion is a history of three or more consecutive spontaneous abortions.

One in four pregnancies end in a spontaneous abortion. Thus by chance alone, it is possible to lose more than three pregnancies but, if these were wanted pregnancies, the psychological stress put upon the couple may warrant further investigations as to the cause, which is rarely found.

Potential Causes

1. Chromosomal: most spontaneous abortions are chromosomally unbalanced.
2. Rhesus isoimmunization.
3. Infection:
    (a) Listeriosis (*Listeria monocytogenes*)
    (b) Toxoplasmosis (*Toxoplasma gondii*)
    (c) Chlamydiosis (*Chlamydia trachomatis*)
    (d) Brucellosis.

4. Abnormal uterine shape: fibroids.
5. Metabolic:
   (a) Renal disease
   (b) Diabetes.
6. Immunological causes (related to the maternal/fetal body host interaction) and the presence of lupus anticoagulant.

Hormonal Causes

1. Hypothyroidism.
2. Progesterone deficiency, although this has never been well documented as a primary cause.

Investigations

1. Chromosomal analysis of both partners.
2. Hysterosalpingogram.
3. Infection antibody screen.
4. Clotting screen to exclude lupus anticoagulant.
5. Tissue typing of both paternal and maternal blood.

Treatment

Thirty years ago diethylstilboestrol (DES) was recommended as treatment and a severe price has been paid by the female offspring, who have a high risk of developing vaginal adenosis and carcinoma of the vagina. The progestogens used then caused masculinization of the female fetus, and had other teratogenic effects with no evidence of therapeutic benefit. There is, therefore, a great danger in treating recurrent abortions with hormones, especially when there is no proven benefit.

Recent work has suggested that sensitizing the mother to the father's white cells may reduce the incidence of recurrent abortion.

Rest in bed in hospital may help pyschologically to relieve the patient's fear and have a good placebo response.

ENDOMETRIOSIS

The relationship between mild endometriosis and infertility is uncertain. It has been suggested that there may be a higher incidence of LUF cycles in endometriotic cycles than in normal cycles; other ovulatory or oocyte abnormalities have been suggested. However, treating mild endometriosis effectively does not appear to improve conception rates. Thus an open mind is needed at present.

19

Fertility Control

INTRODUCTION

Only hormonal methods of fertility control are considered here. The methods that will be considered are:

1. Combined
2. Phasic (biphasic and triphasic)
3. Progestogen only
4. Sequential
5. Postcoital contraception
6. Injectable depot progestogens
7. Medicated IUCD
8. GnRH agonists
9. Prostaglandin termination
10. Antiprogesterones.

Table 19.1 shows the recommended choices of oral contraception. Figure 19.1 shows the factors to be considered in their prescription.

Table 19.1 Choice of oral contraception

Normal women	Phased
Absent minded women	Combined
Smoker over 30 years	Progestogen only
Women over 35 years	Progestogen only
Breakthrough bleeding	Higher dose
Weight gain, depression, loss of libido, acne	Higher oestrogen
Nausea, vertigo, vaginal discharge, breast tenderness	Higher progestogen

METHODS

Combined Oral Contraceptives

These contain oestrogen, usually in the form of ethinyloestradiol or its derivative mestranol, and a progestogen, usually one related

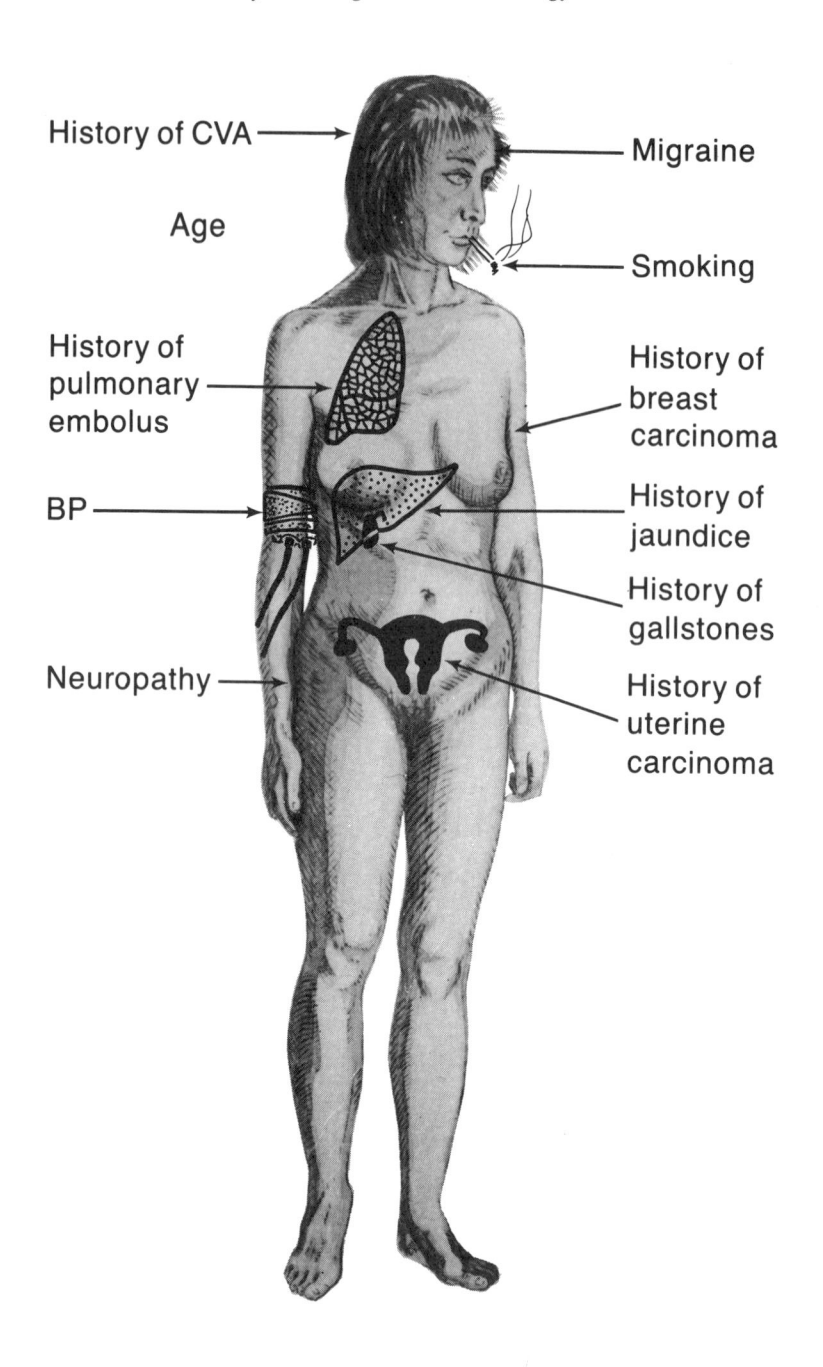

Figure 19.1 Factors to be considered in prescribing oral contraceptives.

to 19-norethisterone. The dose of both remains constant throughout the cycle and they are given for the 21 days with a 7-day break. These are the most commonly prescribed type of pill in the UK.

Their mode of action is to suppress GnRH and thus reduce FSH, preventing the LH surge. The cervical mucus remains thick and the endometrium is affected. Because the FSH is not totally suppressed small ovarian cysts may form, detectable by ultrasound scan.

Phasic Pills

These are designed to mimic the hormonal status of the normal menstrual cycle more closely. The total steroid dose is smaller and they are claimed to have a less adverse effect on blood lipids. They appear to be more effective in controlling bleeding with less breakthrough bleeding. They may be phased with two different doses of progestogen: *biphasic pills* (e.g. Binovum) or with three different doses, the *triphasic pills* (e.g. Logynon, Trinordiol and Trinovum). They do appear to have a reduced margin of error and are more complex to take correctly. Some women claim to develop premenstrual syndrome during the last phase.

Progestogen-only Pills

These must be taken at the same time every day and have a very low margin of error, and are therefore only appropriate for reliable pill-takers. They may cause irregular bleeding or amenorrhoea. Their mode of action appears to be mainly on cervical mucus and by making the endometrium hostile to implantation. They may affect the LH surge. There may be an increased risk of ectopic pregnancy in progestogen-only pill-takers so they are not suitable for women who have had such a pregnancy. They are particularly suitable for women over 35 years, smokers, those in whom there is a relative oestrogen risk or in whom oestrogen is an absolute contraindication.

Sequential Pills

These are no longer used in the UK. Oestrogen was given for 21 days and a progestogen added for a few days at the end of each course.

Postcoital Contraception

This is only effective if used *within 72 hours* of intercourse when high doses of oestrogen can promote a $PGF_2\alpha$ anti-LH effect. Once HCG is produced, this effect is useless to prevent pregnancy. It should only be used once, after which more suitable long-term contraception should be used.

Two tablets of *Ovran 50* or *Eugynon 50* are given and the dose repeated after 12 hours. The patient should be seen again to confirm that this did not fail. If she is pregnant, exposure to the oestrogen or progestogen poses little risk to the fetus at this stage.

Injectable Depot Progestogen

A depot of medroxyprogesterone acetate (Depo-Provera) is most commonly used. It blocks the LH surge but allows some FSH secretion, so endogeneous oestrogen production continues. It is contraceptively effective for about 3 months but may remain in the system for up to 9 months. Irregular bleeding and weight gain are the major disadvantages. It is recommended as a contraceptive after rubella vaccination and while awaiting a negative sperm count postvasectomy.

It can be used as repeated 3 monthly injections but is apt to cause menstrual upsets, so is not routinely recommended. There are reports of increased incidence of mammary cancer in Beagle dogs but close observations of millions of women over 15 years has failed to show an increased risk of breast or uterine cancer.

Medicated IUCD

These are IUCDs which have been coated with a slow release progestogen. They were withdrawn in Great Britain after reports of a high incidence of ectopic pregnancy in users.

GnRH Agonists

By lowering the FSH and LH, GnRH agonists may be contraceptive at some future date. However, to render the patient hypooestrogenic at the same time would leave her exposed to the risk of osteoporosis. This group of substances may prove to be useful contraceptives in time.

Prostaglandin Termination

Termination should not be considered as a method of contraception. However the use of extra- or intra-amniotic prostaglandin have proved to be effective ways of inducing mid-trimester abortions without the same risk to future pregnancies as hysterotomy.

Antiprogesterones

Antiprogesterone agents are now being developed. They may have a role as contraceptive agents. They are also undergoing investigations as a medical method of inducing abortion.

SIDE-EFFECTS OF ORAL CONTRACEPTION

The risks and side-effects will vary with the type of contraceptive pill. In Great Britain the 50 μg oestrogen pills are no longer recommended routinely because they are associated with a higher risk of cardiovascular problems. Oral contraceptives appear to be protective for ovarian carcinoma. Other drugs being taken by the patient may affect hormonal contraception (see Table 19.2).

Table 19.2 Drug interference by hormonal contraceptives

Effect	Drug type	Examples
Reduced contraceptive effect	Antibiotics	Ampicillin
		Rifampicin
	Anticonvulsants	Phenobarbitone
		Phenytoin
	Sedatives	Largactil
		Dichloralphenazone
Reduced drug effect	Tricyclics	Imipramine
		Amitryptiline
	Insulin	
	Anticoagulants	Warfarin

CONTRAINDICATIONS

1. Past history of thrombosis. Cerebral vascular accident.
2. Hypertension.
3. Severe classical migraine.
4. Hyperlipidaemia.
5. Badly controlled diabetes with evidence of neuropathy/retinopathy.
6. Sickle cell disease.

7. Cigarette smoking (if over 30 years).
8. Within 6 months of infectious hepatitis.
9. Cirrhosis.
10. Cholelithiasis.
11. Past history of oestrogen-sensitive cancer (breast or uterus).
12. Recent hydatidiform mole (until HCG levels have returned to normal).
13. Other hormonally sensitive problems such as acute fatty liver of pregnancy and herpes gestationis which are very rare.

Figure 19.2 summarizes the major side-effects of oral contraceptives.

Oestrogen-containing pills should be stopped and alternative contraception used before elective surgery.

WHICH PILL?

Start with a low dose pill. The phased pills have less total steroid and better bleeding control, and are therefore good alternatives on which to start a patient. However, the margin of safety if the patient forgets to take a pill is less and therefore they are not suitable for the slightly absent-minded patient.

In women over 35 years, or smokers of over 30 years, the progestogen-only pill should be considered.

If the patient has breakthrough bleeding, for which other pathology has been excluded, then a higher dose pill should be tried.

Change to a more oestrogenic pill if the patient complains of:

1. Increased weight.
2. Depression/loss of libido.
3. Dry vagina.
4. Acne/greasy skin.

Change to a more progestogenic pill if the patient complains of:

1. Nausea.
2. Dizziness.
3. Vaginal discharge.
4. Breast tenderness.

Figure 19.3 shows the hormone potency balance of the 20 most commonly prescribed oral contraceptives.

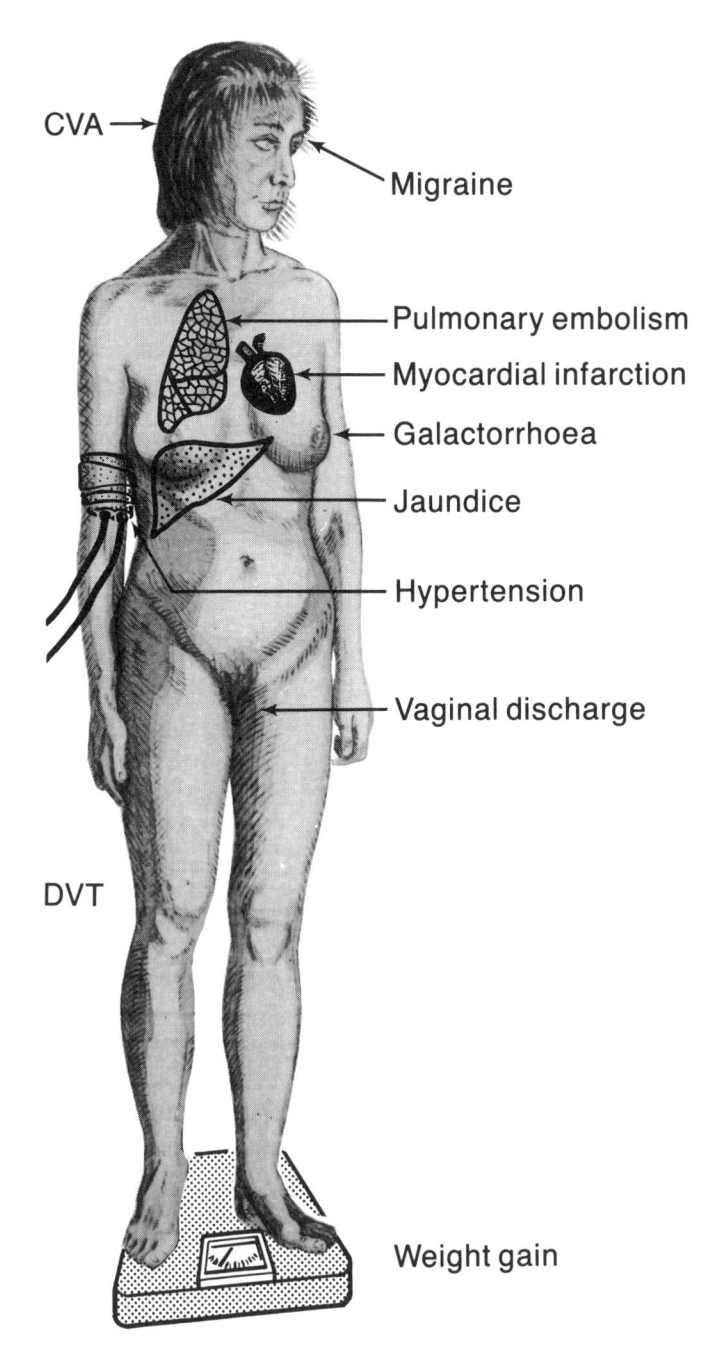

Figure 19.2 Major side-effects of oral contraceptives.

Oestrogen potency
Ethinyloestradiol (μg)

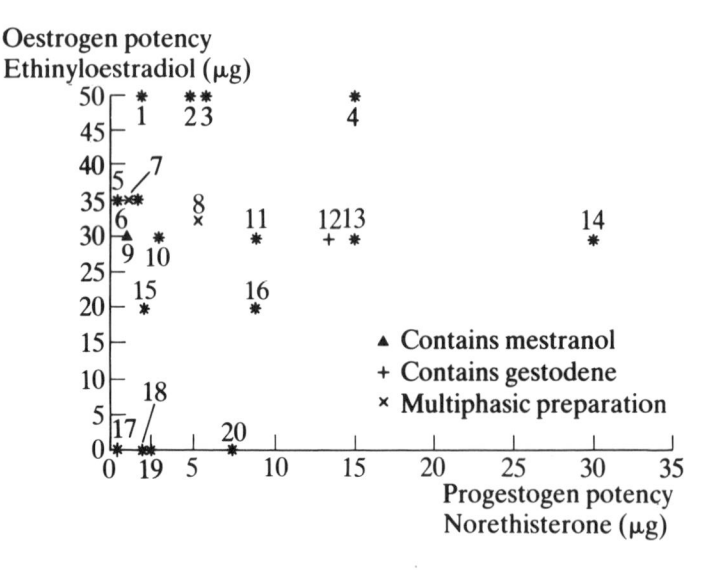

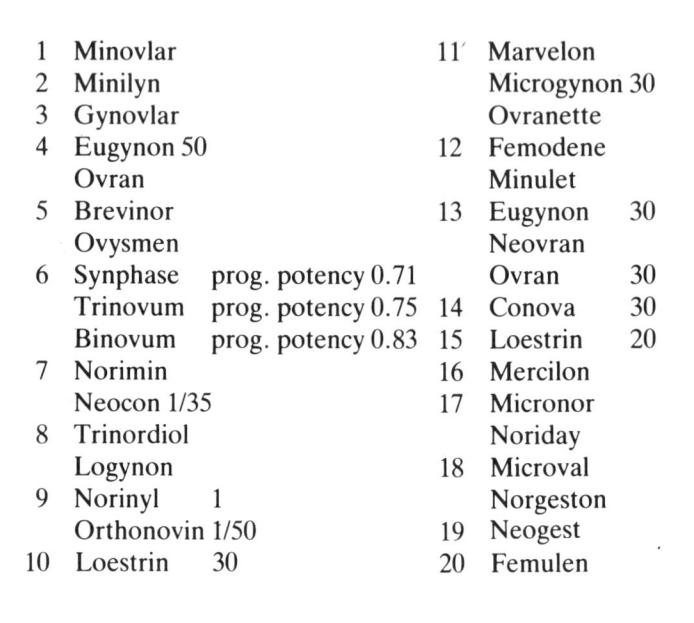

[Scatter plot showing numbered data points 1-20 plotted against Progestogen potency Norethisterone (μg) on x-axis (0-35) and Oestrogen potency on y-axis (0-50). Legend: ▲ Contains mestranol, + Contains gestodene, × Multiphasic preparation]

1	Minovlar	11	Marvelon
2	Minilyn		Microgynon 30
3	Gynovlar		Ovranette
4	Eugynon 50	12	Femodene
	Ovran		Minulet
5	Brevinor	13	Eugynon 30
	Ovysmen		Neovran
6	Synphase prog. potency 0.71		Ovran 30
	Trinovum prog. potency 0.75	14	Conova 30
	Binovum prog. potency 0.83	15	Loestrin 20
7	Norimin	16	Mercilon
	Neocon 1/35	17	Micronor
8	Trinordiol		Noriday
	Logynon	18	Microval
9	Norinyl 1		Norgeston
	Orthonovin 1/50	19	Neogest
10	Loestrin 30	20	Femulen

Figure 19.3 Hormone potency balance.

20

Endocrinology of Pregnancy

INTRODUCTION

As this book concentrates on gynaecological endrocrinology, the endocrinology of pregnancy is only covered briefly. It will not deal with the obstetric management of endocrine disorders. However the golden rule to be observed in all these cases is:

The best possible control should be obtained prior to conception and maintained throughout pregnancy for the best fetal outcome.

Pregnancy is associated with massive changes in hormone levels which are many times greater than the fluctuations found during the menstrual cycle.

While the early conceptus is travelling down the fallopian tube it sends messages to the corpus luteum and endometrium. However against the background of the vast changes in the other hormones, all the mysteries of this process have not yet been unravelled.

THE PLACENTA

This organ produces various proteins present in pregnancy and is involved with the fetus in steroidogenesis. Neither the fetus nor the placenta independently have all the components necessary for steroidogenesis, but together they can and do produce large quantities of steroids. For example, the fetus cannot make progesterone but the placenta can and does so in large quantities.

Progesterone

Progesterone is produced by the corpus luteum and the placenta. Progesterone levels are higher in the luteal phase of ovulatory cycles in which conception has occurred than in cycles in which it did not. All the steroids produced by the feto-placental unit show an S-shaped curve in relation to gestation. Progesterone reaches plasma levels of 200 ng ml^{-1}. Progesterone is obviously involved in changes in the endometrium for implantation and it may also have a role in:

1. Suppression of the maternal immune system to prevent fetal rejection.
2. Providing the fetus with a substrate for other steroids, e.g. corticosteroids.
3. Parturition and the onset of labour.

Oestrogens

While the corpus luteum makes a small amount of oestradiol, oestrogen levels start to rise once the placenta starts to function. During pregnancy the oestrogen found in the largest amounts is oestriol, which is a relatively weak oestrogen. It is first detected at 9 weeks, because it needs the fetal adrenal to first produce the necessary precursor, dehydroepiandrosterone sulphate (DHAS). The levels rise until 31 weeks and then plateau until 35 weeks when the levels again rise. By the end of pregnancy oestriol levels are a thousand times higher than the non-pregnant levels. The role of oestriol in pregnancy is not clear as very low oestriol levels are found in the condition of placental sulphatase deficiency but the fetus is healthy and of normal size.

Human Chorionic Gonadotrophin

Human chorionic gonadotrophin (HCG) is very similar to LH but has a longer half-life than LH. The corpus luteum needs HCG stimulation in order to continue, thus HCG is one of the first hormones produced during pregnancy. The levels increase to a maximum of 100 000 units at about 10 weeks and then regress again to about 10 000 units by 20 weeks, remaining at this level until term. HCG is involved in steroidogenesis in early pregnancy. Clinically, HCG is used in routine pregnancy tests. In ectopic pregnancy the levels may be lower than anticipated by the length of amenorrhoea. An ultrasensitive pregnancy test will be positive at 25 or 50 units but the patient may have a negative test at 500 units and this will imply either an ectopic pregnancy, a very early pregnancy or the falling levels after a complete abortion. In trophoblastic disease there are very high levels and HCG can be used as a marker to confirm full treatment of the disease. It can also be used as a tumour marker for some ovarian tumours. A false-positive pregnancy test may be due to heavy proteinuria, haematuria or a high LH at the menopause.

Other proteins made by the placenta and referred to by their initials may have a role as tests of fetal well-being:

1. Pregnancy Associated Plasma Protein A (PAPP A)
2. Human Placental Lactogen (HPL)
3. Pregnancy specific β_1 glycoprotein (SP1)
4. Pregnancy Associated Plasma Protein B (PAPP B)
5. Pregnancy Associated Plasma Protein C (PAPP C)
6. Placental Protein 5 (PP5).

STAGES OF PREGNANCY

Early Pregnancy

The signs and symptoms of pregnancy are related to the changing hormone levels (see Figure 20.1). The high oestrogen or HCG levels may induce the symptoms of nausea and vomiting, as well as breast enlargement and tenderness.

Sexual Differentiation

In the absence of any positive stimulation the fetus develops as phenotypically female. Both X chromosomes are usually needed for ovarian development. The development of the HY antigen and appropriate androgen receptors are necessary for the testes to form. Once formed they produce anti-müllerian factor (AMF) to induce regression of the müllerian system in the male. This occurs between 7 and 16 weeks. During this time the fetus is very sensitive to exogenous hormone administration, e.g. testosterone or its derivatives (most progestogens) which virilize the female fetus.

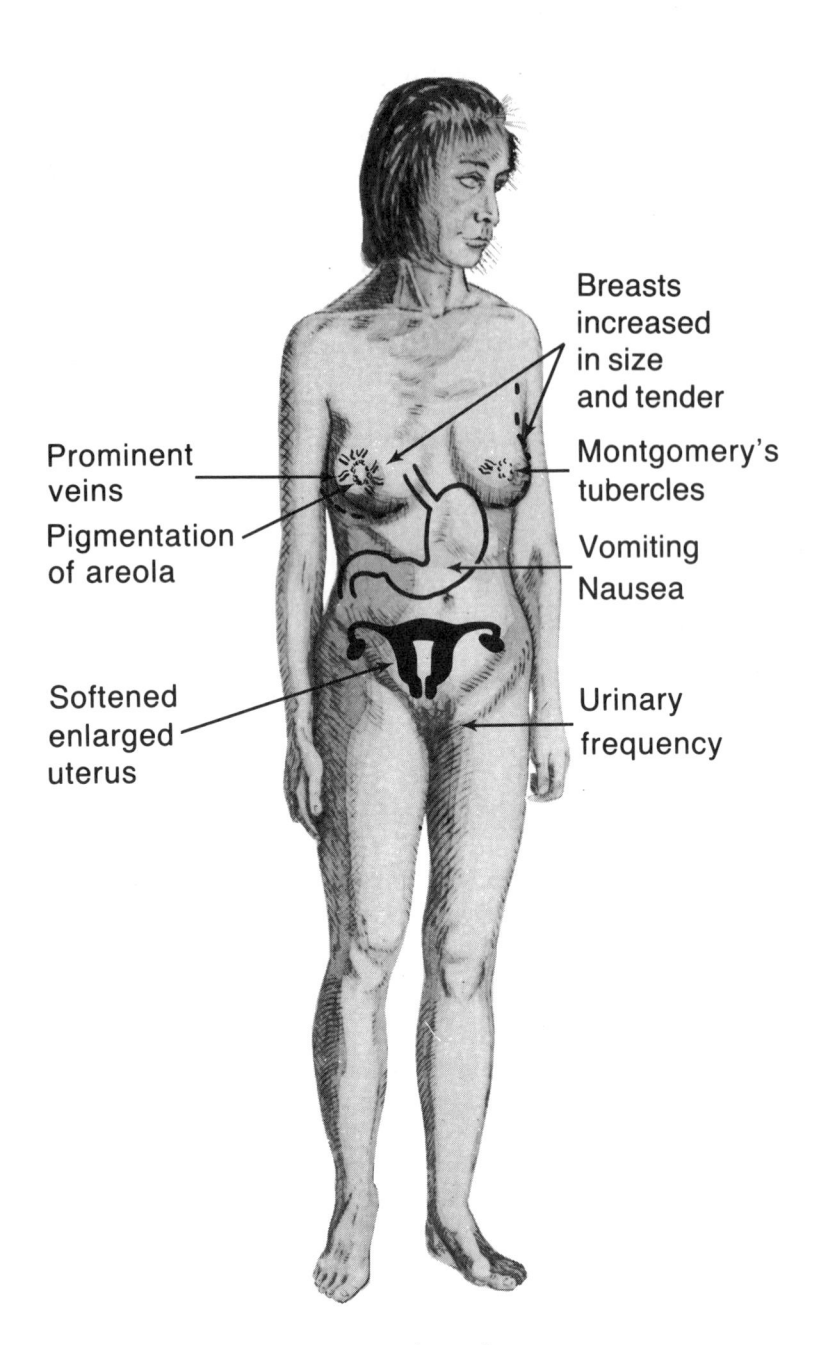

Figure 20.1 Early signs of pregnancy.

Onset of Labour

The mechanisms involved in the onset of human labour are not yet fully understood. Much of the research in this area has been performed on chronically catheterized sheep in whom the fetal pituitary is the prime initiator. However, in humans, 41% of anencephalic fetuses deliver before 38 weeks, thus the mechanisms for the onset of labour must be different. Of the many hormones involved it seems that oestrogen and progesterone have a role in initiating a rise in oxytocin and prostaglandins.

21

The Menopause

Definitions
The menopause is the time of cessation of the menses.

The climacteric is the period on either side of the menopause lasting many months or years during which ovarian oestrogen starts to fail and ultimately ceases.

INTRODUCTION

The average age of menopause in Great Britain is 51 years; a late menarche may correlate with early menopause. During the climacteric there is a gradual change by the body to using oestrone, formed by peripheral convertion of androstenedione, rather than oestradiol produced by the ovary. This oestrogen withdrawal results in raised FSH and LH levels.

RESULTS OF OESTROGEN WITHDRAWAL

Menstrual Changes

Anovulation usually precedes the menopause by one or two years, and gradually the menstrual loss decreases. The menopause may come in one of three ways, or a combination of these.

1. Increasingly shorter duration and scantier loss lasting 1 or 2 days, and then only a few hours, but coming at the time of an expected menstruation.

2. Missed menstruation, followed by a return of menstruation for a few cycles, but each menstruation lasting the normal 5–7 days and coming at the time of expected menstruation.
3. Sudden end with no history of missed menstruation or shorter duration. This type occurs when there has been a sudden change in lifestyle, e.g. moving house or bereavement.

Physical Changes

These include:

1. Thinning skin, causing wrinkles.
2. Thinning vagina.
3. Increased pH in the vagina which leads to a change in the bacterial flora of the vagina. These changes result in the tendency to atrophic vaginitis and increased tendency to 'frictional' dyspareunia.
4. Atrophy of the breasts.
5. Atrophy of the labia.
6. Reduction in size of the uterus.
7. Pelvic floor muscle laxity which causes the increased incidence of prolapse.
8. Thinning of the bladder and urethral epithelium which may cause an increase in urinary symptoms of frequency and urgency.

The most common menopausal symptoms are shown in Figure 21.1.

Vasomotor Changes

The patient experiences *hot flushes* which tend to start in the chest, spread up to the head and neck, and then to the rest of the body. They give rise to a transient sensation lasting only a few minutes. If a patient says the flush lasts for 30 minutes on each occasion, consider other causes of flushes, e.g. carcinoid tumour or PUO. Flushes may be visible or invisible to the observer. Increased sweats usually occur at night; the woman awakes drenched in sweat and she may have to change her nightclothes.

Osteoporosis

The bone increases in porosity and brittleness in postmenopausal

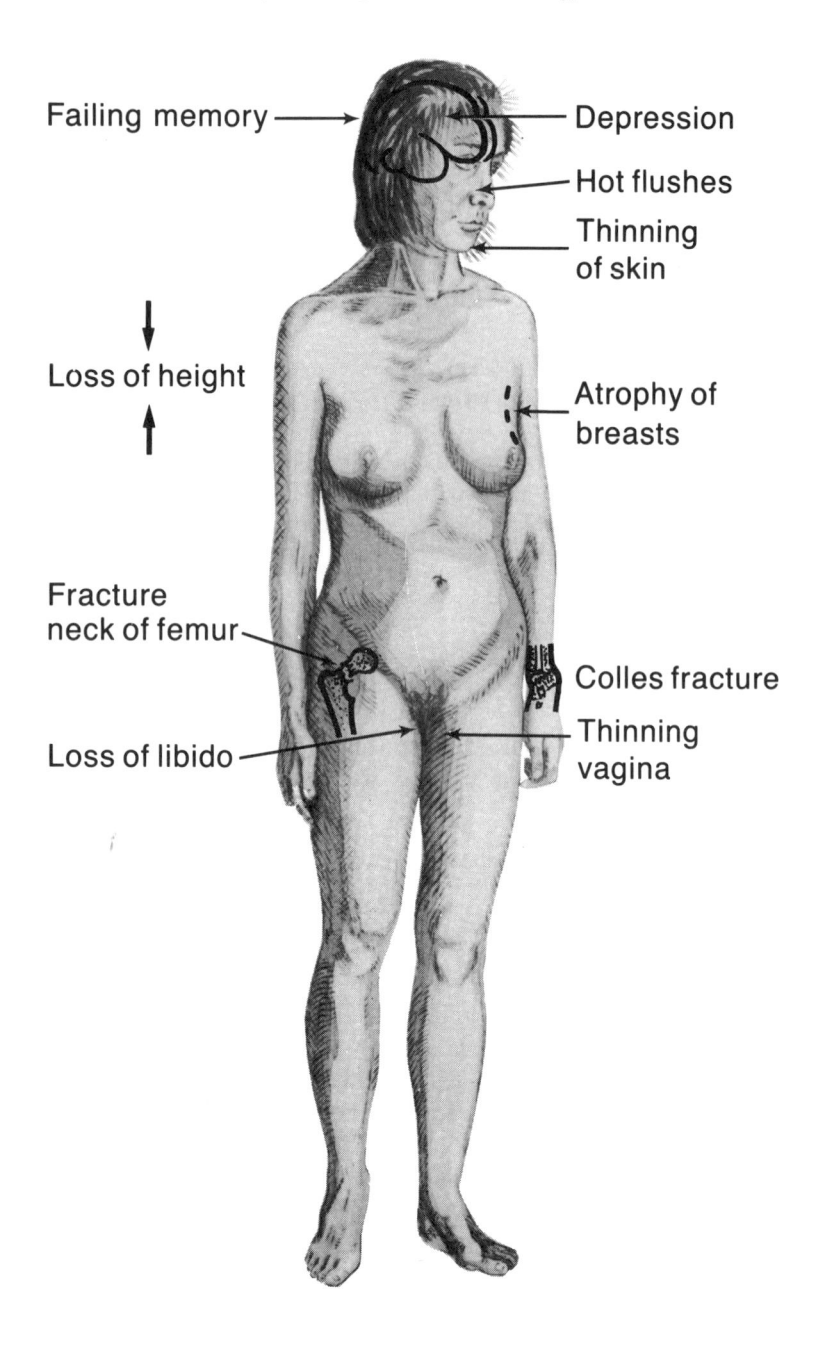

Figure 21.1 Menopausal symptoms.

women, leading to a high incidence of fractures. Fractured head of femur tends to occur in 'little old ladies': 'little' as they do not have much body fat and their height has been reduced due to fracture and compression of the vertebrae; 'old' because they are post-menopausal; and 'ladies' because the development of osteoporosis starts much later in men.

There is a high incidence of spinal compression which results in a shrinkage in height in postmenopausal women. These changes are related to the effect of oestrogen withdrawal on calcium metabolism and are also observed in the young woman castrated at an early age. Postmenopausal osteoporosis is responsible for a large number of orthopaedic admissions and elimination of the problems would save both unnecessary suffering and hospital resources.

Psychological Disturbances

1. Depressed mood.
2. Insomnia, which is not helped by sweats waking the patient at night.
3. Failing memory.
4. Loss of libido.

Other Changes

1. A rise in the levels of cholesterol, triglycerides and phospholipids.
2. Increase in the incidence of coronary arterial disease.

EXAMINATION

1. Check thyroid.
2. Thinning of skin on arms and wrinkles on face.
3. Atrophic breasts.
4. Vagina: pale, dry, thin and atrophic.
5. Cervix, small and firm.

INVESTIGATIONS

1. Raised FSH and LH.

TREATMENT

The treatment of menopausal symptoms is summarized in Figure 21.2. Note that any treatment should be stopped after 6 months to see if the symptoms have settled, and then restarted if necessary.

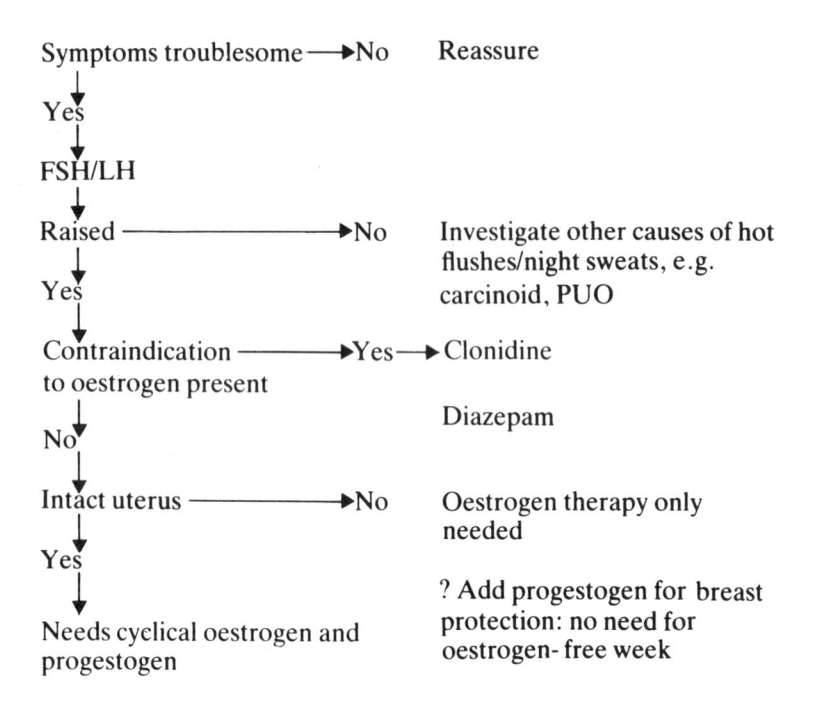

Symptoms troublesome → No   Reassure
↓
Yes
↓
FSH/LH
↓
Raised ──────────→ No   Investigate other causes of hot
↓   flushes/night sweats, e.g.
Yes   carcinoid, PUO
↓
Contraindication ─────→ Yes → Clonidine
to oestrogen present
↓   Diazepam
No
↓
Intact uterus ─────────→ No   Oestrogen therapy only
↓   needed
Yes
↓   ? Add progestogen for breast
Needs cyclical oestrogen and   protection: no need for
progestogen   oestrogen-free week

Figure 21.2 The management of the climacteric.

Non-hormonal

Simple measures such as the avoidance of hot drinks and sudden changes in temperature will help. The hot flushes and night sweats may be helped by clonidine or propranolol. Anti-depressants may help the psychological symptoms. Adequate calcium intake in the diet and regular exercise reduce the development of osteoporosis.

Hormonal

OESTROGENS

If a woman has a uterus she *must* also have cyclical progestogen. Oestrogens, which are easily converted into oestrone, are recommended. Oestrone sulphate (Harmogen) or oestradiol valerate (Progynova) are favoured. Conjugated equine oestrogen (Premarin) used to be popular, but it contains many different steroids which tend to have more effect on the clotting factors and the new preparations are probably superior.

The latest of these are skin patches providing a continuous release of oestradiol giving good blood levels while avoiding the 'first pass' through the liver, and thus reducing the metabolic side-effects of taking oestrogens. This route may become the common way to give hormones that are absorbable transdermally.

PROGESTOGENS

Recent evidence suggests that norethisterone is probably the best progestogen for preventing endometrial hyperplasia and reducing the risk of developing carcinoma of the endometrium, a risk present in unopposed oestrogen therapy. Ideally, norethisterone should be given in a low dose for 12 days. Unfortunately low dose norethisterone is not currently available in this country. Norgestrel is commonly used in combined packs of menopausal treatments.

Women who have had a hysterectomy do not need the progestogen to protect their endometrium; whether the progestogen also plays a role in protecting the breast from breast cancer is still debatable.

Progestogens also slow down bone loss.

22

Drugs Used in Gynaecological Endocrinology

INTRODUCTION

The purpose of this section is to help the SHO left at the far end of the clinic with a queue of 'return patients' waiting to be seen. The majority of these patients will be suffering from one of the problems discussed in this book, while the more senior doctors are seeing and assessing the new patients. It is not an attempt to give a complete list of all possible treatments but merely a guide.

OESTROGENS

Uses

1. Hormonal contraception.
2. Menopausal 'replacement' therapy.

Contraindications

Absolute

1. Oestrogen-sensitive cancer — endometrial or breast.
2. Past history of thromboembolism.

3. Previous cerebral vascular accident.
4. Chronic liver disease.

Relative

1. Severe (crescendo) migraine.
2. Hypertension.
3. Hyperlipidaemia.
4. Severe unstable diabetes.
5. Cigarette smoking.
6. Grossly obese.
7. Sickle cell anaemia.
8. Within 6 months of hepatitis.
9. Cholelithiasis.

Metabolic Changes

These are summarised in Table 22.1

Table 22.1 Metabolic changes induced by oestrogen administration

Liver function tests	Transaminases increase
	Albumin increases
	Blood sugar increases
Clotting factors	Antithrombin III increases
	Fibrinolysis increases
	Platelet aggregation increases
	Blood viscosity increases
Hormones	Insulin increases
	Growth hormone increases
	Thyroxine increases
	Prolactin increases
	Binding globulins increase
Renal	Renin substrate increases
	Angiotensin II increases

Side-effects

1. Carcinoma of the endometrium/irregular uterine bleeding. A progestogen *must* also be used if the patient has her uterus.
2. Thromboembolism and cerebral vascular accident.
3. Myocardial infarction.
4. Fluid retention.

5. Headache.
6. Nausea.
7. Galactorrhoea.

Forms Available

HORMONAL CONTRACEPTION

See page 101.

1. Start on a low dose phasic pill.

MENOPAUSAL THERAPY

1. Piperazine oestrone sulphate (Harmogen) 1.5–4.5 mg daily. *Advantages:* it is the nearest 'natural' oestrogen to the body's natural pool of oestrone, and has little effect on clotting factors. *Disadvantage:* no pack available with a combined progestogen.
2. Oestradiol valerate (Progynova) 1–2 mg. *Advantage:* it is readily converted to oestrone and a pack with added progestogen (Cycloprogynova) is available. *Disadvantage:* the progestogen used is not ideal.
3. Conjugated equine oestrogens (Premarin) 0.625–1.25 mg. *Advantage:* combined pack (Prempak C) has a long course of progestogen. *Disadvantage:* it contains many different steroids (approximately 20), has greater effects on clotting factors, including equilin which is another carcinogen to the endometrium, and the progestogen is norgestrel.
4. Oestrogen skin patches. *Advantage:* avoids 'first pass' through the liver, so there are fewer metabolic side-effects. *Disadvantage:* some people develop an allergy to the adhesive. The patches should be changed twice a week.
5. Oestrogen cream may be used in atrophic vaginitis, but because there is systemic absorption by this route, the amount of which may vary, it should only be used judiciously. Oestriol cream and pessaries are now available. An oestriol is a weaker oestrogen and is not as well absorbed from the vagina, but it is equally effective in atrophic vaginitis and should now be considered as first line of treatment, with dienoestrol cream as second choice.

PROGESTERONE

Uses

Premenstrual syndrome (see page 84). Progesterone preparations available at present are poorly absorbed orally but can be administered by IM injection, vaginally or rectally; for example, progesterone suppositories (Cyclogest) 400 mg bd from day 14 until the onset of menstruation. The dose of the suppositories may be increased to six times a day if necessary. A nulliparous patient may need a lower dose. Progesterone is usually well tolerated but irregular bleeding can occur.

PROGESTOGENS

Uses

1. *Prevention of endometrial hyperplasia.* Progestogen is given when oestrogen is needed and the woman has a uterus. There is less chance of patient error if a combined pack is used.
2. *Addition of progestogen to a course of oestrogen.* Theoretically low dose norethisterone 20 µg for 12 days is sufficient; unfortunately no such preparation is available at the moment. The best option may therefore be Noriday or Micronor, which both have 35 µg in each tablet, used for the last 14 days of a 21-day course of oestrogen.
3. *Cycle control.* In menorrhagia, norethisterone 5 mg bd from day 19 to day 26. If this does not prevent irregular bleeding the course may be extended from days 5–21. If the menses are still too heavy 5 mg tds may be used. If there are side-effects try dydrogesterone 10 mg bd.
4. *Progestogen challenge test.* Medroxyprogesterone acetate (Provera) 10 mg bd for 5 days, pregnancy having been excluded.
5. *Premenstrual syndrome.* Dydrogesterone 10 mg days 14–28. Side-effects: nausea, migraine and water retention with progest*ogens* but not reported with progest*erone*.

Contraindications

1. Impaired liver function.
2. Breast carcinoma.
3. Hyperlipidaemia.
4. Masculinization of the female fetus with progesto*gens*, but not with pure natural progest*erone*.

Caution should be used in prescribing these drugs to women with a past history of thromboembolism and hypertension.

Forms Available

1. Norethisterone
2. Medroxyprogesterone acetate
3. Dydrogesterone

TESTOSTERONE

Uses

1. Loss of libido in the menopause.
2. Pruritus vulvae.

Contraindications

1. Pregnancy.
2. Liver disease.

Side-effects

1. Virilization.
2. Cholestatic jaundice.

Forms Available

In the treatment of loss of libido in the climacteric, an implant (100 mg) may be inserted and renewed every 6 to 9 months as required. For pruritus vulvae, a 2% cream applied topically daily may help in chronic vulval dystrophy.

FSH

This is available both in a pure form (Metrodin) and combined with LH in the form of 'Pergonal' injections (FSH 75 units, LH 24 units). This should only be given under close supervision with monitoring of oestrogens and/or follicular development. It should only be used after failure to induce ovulation with an anti-oestrogen for superovulation.

Contraindications

Inability to monitor effectively.

Side-effects

Hyperstimulation syndrome. This can be so severe, with the sudden formation of massive ovarian cysts, that the patient suffers a serious fluid imbalance and electrolyte disturbance, and develops a disseminated intravascular coagulopathy. Death caused by inappropriate dosage has been reported.

LH

Luteinizing hormone is usually given as HCG. It is used to induce ovulation, either after priming with clomiphene, tamoxifen or Pergonal. Repeated injections may be given for the continuance of pregnancy.

GnRH

1. This can be administered via a pump in pulses for ovulation induction.
2. Agonists of GnRH may be used for their ability to down regulate the receptor; they can 'switch off' the pituitary, and thus LH and FSH release. This may be useful in treating endometriosis and fibroids. They can also be used for ovulation

induction in *in vitro* fertilization where they may help to allow multiple follicles to develop.

ANTI-OESTROGENS

Use

Clomiphene is the most commonly used anti-oestrogen for ovulation induction. Dosage starts at 50 mg on days 2–6, and if anovulation persists it should be increased up to 200 mg daily.

Side-effects

1. Hot flushes.
2. Nausea.
3. Ovarian cyst development.
4. Risk of multiple pregnancy.

BROMOCRIPTINE

Uses

1. Hyperprolactinaemia.
2. To suppress lactation.

Dosage

For hyperprolactinaemia, a dose of 2.5 mg daily is given and increased until the patient is euprolactinaemic, then decreased gradually.

To suppress lactation, 2.5 mg bd is given for 10 days. This is only appropriate in women who have had a stillbirth or neonatal death.

Side-effects

1. Nausea and fainting, which can be eased by taking the tablets with food immediately before retiring.
2. Postural hypotension.
3. Sweating.

DANAZOL

Uses

1. As an 'antigonadatrophin' for endometriosis.
2. As a progestogen for menorrhagia and mastitis.

Dosage

Danazol will render the patient amenorrhoeic at doses of 200 mg tds or qds and is used to treat endometriosis. It may also shrink fibroids. At lower dosages its powerful progestogenic properties may be used in the treatment of menorrhagia or mastalgia: 100 mg daily may be enough, reducing on alternate days after 3 months and then stopping treatment.

Contraindications

1. Pregnancy.
2. Renal impairment.

Side-effects

1. Water retention and weight gain.
2. Acne.
3. Hirsutism.
4. Rashes.
5. Deepening of the voice (if this occurs the treatment should be stopped *immediately*).

CYPROTERONE ACETATE

Uses

1. Hirsutism.
2. Acne.

Dosage

Cyproterone acetate is an anti-androgen. It may be given at a low dose in either of the following two forms.
1. *Diane,* which is useful in acne, comes as a form of oral contraceptive in a combined preparation with 2 mg cyproterone acetate.
2. *Cyproterone acetate* 50 mg on days 5–15 and *ethinyl oestradiol* 30 mg on days 5–26.

It takes about 9 months to notice an improvement in hirsutism. The regime is designed in the reverse way because cyproterone acetate remains in the fat for a long time and so needs to be administered early in the cycle. The addition of an oestrogen not only makes the regime contraceptive, but also helps with cycle control and has beneficial effects on hirsutism.

Contraindications

1. Pregnancy — it will cause feminization of the male fetus.
2. Liver disease.
3. Adrenal suppression.

PROSTAGLANDIN SYNTHETASE INHIBITORS

Uses

1. Dysmenorrhoea.
2. Menorrhagia.

Dosage

Mefenamic acid 250 mg qds to 500 mg tds on days 1–3.

Contraindications

1. Inflammatory bowel disease.
2. Peptic ulceration.
3. Renal impairment.
4. Liver impairment.

Side-effects

1. Skin rashes.
2. Diarrhoea.
3. Bronchospasm.

Prostaglandin may be used for termination of pregnancy (see page 104)

Bibliography

ABPI (1988). *ABPI Data Sheet Compendium 1988–1989*. London: ABPI.

Besser, G.M. and Culdworth, A.G. (1987). *Clinical Endocrinology — An Illustrated Text*. London: Chapman & Hall.

Dalton, K. (1984). *The Premenstrual Syndrome and Progesterone Therapy*, 2nd edn. London: Heinemann.

Dewhurst, J. (1985). *Female Puberty and its Abnormalities*. Edinburgh: Churchill Livingstone.

Fuchs, F. and Klopper, A. (1983). *Endocrinology of Pregnancy*, 3rd edn. Philadelphia, PA: Harper & Row

Ingbar, S.H. and Brauerman, L.E. (1986). *Werner's The Thyroid; A Fundamental and Clinical Text*, 5th edn. Philadelphia, PA: J.B. Lippincott.

Insler, V. and Lunenfield, B. (Eds) (1985). *Infertility: Male and Female*. Edinburgh: Churchill Livingstone.

Rosenwaks, Z., Benjamin, F. and Stone, M.L. (1987). *Gynecology: Principles and Practices*. New York: Macmillan.

Shearman, R. (1985). *Clinical Reproductive Endocrinology*. Edinburgh: Churchill Livingstone.

Speroff, L., Glass, R.H. and Kase, N.G. (1983). *Clinical Gynecological Endocrinology and Infertility*, 3rd edn. Baltimore, MD: Williams & Wilkins.

Stanhope, R., Adams, J. and Brook, C.G.D. (1985). Disturbances of puberty, *Clinics in Obstetrics and Gynaecology*, **12**(3), 575–577.

Index

Abortion, recurrent 98-99
Acidophils 5
Acne 64, 80-81, 85-86, 101, 127-128
Acromegaly 21, 55, 59, 64, 79
ACTH 3-5, 7, 10, 16-19, 34, 79
Addison's syndrome 17, 66, 94
Adenergic receptors, alpha and beta 18
Adenomyosis, see Endometriosis
ADH, see Antidiuretic hormone
Adrenal gland 7, 10, 15-18
Adrenal tumour 49-51, 59, 79, 94
Adrenalin 17
Aldosterone 15-16
Amenorrhoea 22, 32, 48, 57-66, 95-96, 110, 127
AMF, see Anti-Mullerian factor
AMP, see Cyclic AMP
Anaemia 69
Androgen insensitivity, see Testicular feminisation
Androgens 10-11, 15-16, 29-30, 79, 124
Androstendione 9-10, 14, 16-17, 21, 59, 61, 82
Anorexia nervosa 58, 65, 77, 93
Anosmia 58, 63
Anovulation 22, 93-98, 114
Anti-androgen 49, 83
Antibiotics 105
Anticoagulants 105

Anticonvulsants 105
Antidiuretic hormone 8
Antigonadotrophin 49, 127
Anti-Mullerian factor 111
Anti-oestrogens 65-66, 96-97, 126
Antiprogesterone 101, 105
Asherman's syndrome 58, 65
Azoospermia 92

Basophils 5
Binding assay 35-36
Biphasic pill 101, 103
Bone 9, 13-15, 115-117
Breast 43, 45, 53-56
  atrophy of 80-81, 115-116
  carcinoma of 55, 101-103, 119-120, 124
  development of 43-45
Bromocriptine 55-56, 60, 96, 98, 126
Brucellosis 98

Calcium 13-15, 118
Calcium antagonists 75-76
Calcitonin 13-15
Chlamydiosis 98
Cholesterol 28
Chorioepithelioma 49-50
Chromophobes 5
Chromosomes 50, 57, 98-99
Climacteric 68, 114-120, 122, 124
CLIP, see Corticotrophic intermediate lobe protein
Clitoris, enlargement of 64, 80, 81

Clomiphene 66, 96-98, 125-126
Clonidine 118
Congenital adrenal hyperplasia 31, 50-52, 59, 66, 79, 94
Contraception 69, 76, 101-108
Corpus luteum 6, 9-10, 38-40
Corticosterone 17, 79, 110
Corticotrophic intermediate lobe protein 7, 26
Corticotrophin releasing hormone (CRH) 3-4, 7
Cortisol 15, 33
Cortisol binding globulin 10, 17, 24, 121
Cortisone 17
CRH, see Corticotrophin releasing hormone
Cushing's syndrome 21, 34, 59, 66, 79, 94
Cyclic AMP 23
Cyclofenil 97
Cyproterone acetate 49, 83, 128

Danazol 47, 49, 56, 71, 73, 75, 90, 127
Dehydroepiandrosterone 10-11, 16-17, 45
Dehydroepiandrosterone sulphate 110
Delayed puberty 50-52, 65
Dexamethasone 83
Dexamethasone suppression test 33, 82
Depression 68-70, 85, 90, 101, 106, 116-117
Diabetes 99, 121
Diethylstilboestrol 99
Dihydrotestosterone 10, 24
Dopamine 3, 6-7
Dydrogesterone 71, 73, 89, 123-124
Dysfunctional uterine bleeding 67-73, 76, 123, 127-128
Dysmenorrhoea 74-76, 90, 128
  congestive 74
  spasmodic 74

Ectopic pregnancy 103, 110, 111
Endometrial carcinoma 22, 67-68, 103, 119-122
Endometrial proteins 41-42
Endometriosis 67-69, 75, 93, 99, 127
Endometrium 9-10, 39-42
Endorphins 7, 19, 58, 88
Enkephalins 19
Epilepsy 86-87
Exercise related amenorrhoea 58, 65-66
Exophalamus 64

Fat 21-22, 60-61
Feedback, hormonal 24-25
Fibroids 67-70, 76, 99
Flushes, hot 63, 69, 115-116, 126
Follicle 9, 19, 37-40
FSH 1, 4-7, 9-11, 19, 23-24, 26, 32, 36-39, 45, 47, 51, 59, 63, 71, 82, 92, 96, 103, 114, 117, 125

Galactorrhoea 53, 63-64, 95, 107, 122, 126
GAP, see Gonadotrophin associated protein
GH, see Growth hormone
GHRH, see Growth hormone releasing hormone
Glucocorticoid 16-17
GnRH, see Gonadotrophin associated releasing hormone
Gonadal angenesis/dysgenesis 51, 58
Gonadotrophin associated protein 6-7
Gonadotrophin associated releasing hormone 1, 3-4, 6-7, 23, 38, 47, 51, 58, 60, 103, 125
Gonadotrophin associated releasing hormone

Index

agonist test 32, 51
Gonadotrophin associated releasing hormone agonists 49, 66, 73, 101, 104
Gonadotrophin stimulation therapy 96–97, 125
Granulosa cell 37, 40
Growth hormone 3–7, 19, 121
Growth hormone releasing hormone 7

Hair
  axillary 45–46, 64, 77, 78
  pubic 45–46, 64, 77–78, 81
HCG, see Human chorionic gonadotrophin
Headache 85, 122
Hirsutism 22, 49, 59–60, 63, 77–83, 95, 127–128
Hot flushes 63, 69, 115–116, 126
17-HP, see 17-Hydroxyprogesterone
HSGs, see Hysterosalpingograms 93, 95, 99
Human chorionic gonadotrophin 6, 40, 97, 103, 106, 110–111, 125
Hydatidiform moles 106
17-Hydroxyprogesterone 59, 63, 82
Hyperprolactinaemia 54–55, 59, 65–66, 79, 88, 94, 98, 126
Hyperstimulation syndrome 97, 125
Hypertension 102, 105, 107, 121, 124
Hyperthyroidism 12, 32–33, 59, 66, 68, 94
Hypogonadotrophic hypogonadism 52, 97
Hypothalamus 1–2, 4–5, 37, 50–51, 58, 60–61, 93
Hypothyroidism 12, 21, 32–33, 49–50, 55, 59, 63, 66, 68–69, 79, 94, 96, 99
Hysterectomy 72–73, 119
Hysterosalpingograms 93, 95, 99

Implantation 41, 92, 103
In vitro fertilization (IVF) 66, 97–98, 126
Infertility 42, 91–100
Inhibin 10–11, 61, 92
Intrauterine contraceptive devices 67–70, 76, 101, 104
IUDs, see Intrauterine contraceptive devices
IVF, see In vitro fertilization

Kallman's syndrome 52, 58
Klinefelter's syndrome 50, 52, 57

Lactation 54, 57
LH, see Luteinizing hormone
Libido, loss of 79, 101, 106, 116, 124
Lipotrophin 3–5, 7, 19
Listeriosis 98
Lisuride 98
LUFS, see Luteinized unruptured follicle syndrome
Lupus anticoagulant 99
Luteinized unruptured follicle syndrome 34, 40, 94, 96, 100
Luteinizing hormone 1, 3–7, 10–11, 19, 23, 32, 38–39, 45, 47, 51, 59, 63, 65, 71, 82, 92–93, 96, 103, 114, 117, 125

McCune-Albright syndrome 49–50
Magnesium 88
Masculinisation 63, 124
Mastalgia 55–56, 85–86, 101, 111–112, 127

Median eminence 1–3
Medroxyprogesterone acetate
 33, 49, 104, 123
Mefanamic acid 73
Melonocyte stimulating
 hormone releasing
 hormone (MSHRH) 3–4
Menarche 43, 45, 48, 50,
 63, 114
 delayed 50–52
Menopause 53–54, 57, 68,
 114–120, 122, 124
Menorrhagia 47, 67–73,
 123, 127–128
Menstrual cycle 37–42
MFO, see Multifollicular
 ovary syndrome
Migraine 86–87, 102, 105,
 107, 121
Mineralocorticoids 15–16
MSHRH, see Melonocyte
 stimulating hormone
 releasing hormone
Multifollicular ovary
 syndrome 48, 58, 62
Myomectomy 72

Neurophysin 7
Norethisterone 56, 71, 73,
 119, 123–124
19–Norethisterone 101

Obesity 21–22, 58, 60, 121
Oestradiol 9, 23–25, 29,
 39–41, 47, 60–61, 71,
 128
Oestriol 9, 38, 110
Oestrogen 4, 6, 9, 11, 15,
 20, 21–22, 30, 37, 51,
 55, 79, 110, 113, 114,
 117, 119–122, 125
Oestrone 9, 21, 30, 119,
 122
Oligomenorrhoea 63, 95
Oligospermia 92
Oocyte 9, 37–38, 97
Oral contraception 54, 75,
 83, 94, 101–108, 122
Osteoporosis 54, 66, 104,
 115–118
Ovarian tumour 49–52, 59,
 68, 79

Ovulation 34, 38–40, 92–93
Ovum 8
Oxytocinon 7–8, 19, 113

Parathormone 13–15
Parathyroid 13
Paraventricular nucleus 1–
 2, 7
PCI, see Prostacyclin
PCO, see Polycystic ovarian
 syndrome
Pelvic inflammatory disease
 67–68, 76
Peptide histidine
 isolencine (PHI) 6–7
Pergonal 97–98, 125
PG, see Prostaglandin
PGSI, see Prostaglandin
 synthetase inhibitors
PID, see Pelvic
 inflammatory disease
PIF, see Prolactin
 inhibiting factor
Pineal gland 3–4
Pituitary gland 1–2, 5, 8,
 37, 50, 58–61, 66, 79,
 94
Placenta 109
PND, see Postnatal
 depression
Polycystic ovarian syndrome
 21–22, 59–62, 65–66,
 68, 79, 82–83, 94, 96
Postcoital bleeding 69, 71
Postcoital contraception
 101, 103–104
Postcoital test 93, 95
Postnatal depression 84
Preantral follicle 37
Precocious puberty 4, 48·
 50
Pregnancy 53–54, 57, 109–
 113, 127–128
Pregnenolone 28, 30
Premature ejaculation 92
Premature menopause, see
 Premature ovarian
 failure
Premature ovarian failure
 59, 65–66, 94, 96
Premenstrual syndrome 55,
 84–90, 123

Progesterone 4, 6, 9–10, 23, 29, 38–41, 47, 71, 87, 89, 95, 96, 99, 101, 103–104, 110, 113, 123
Progestogen 49, 51, 99, 101, 111, 119, 121–124, 127
Progestogen challenge test 34, 63, 123
Progestogen only pill 101, 103
Prolactin 3–4, 6–7, 19, 23, 53–56, 58, 63, 65–66, 82, 121
Prolactin inhibiting factor 6
Prolactin releasing factor 6
Prolactin secreting adenoma 55, 58
Pro-opiomelanocortin 7, 19, 26
Prostacyclin 19
Prostaglandin 19–20, 38, 40–41, 71, 74–75, 88, 103, 113
Prostaglandin synthetase inhibitors 71–72, 75–76, 90, 128
Prostaglandin termination 101, 104, 129
Protein binding assay 35
Protein kinase 24
Puberty 43–53, 68, 80
Pyridoxine 88, 90

Radioimmunassay 35
Resistant ovary syndrome, 59, 65–66, 94, 96
RIA, see Radioimmunassay
Rubella 95, 104

Sex hormone binding globulin (SHBG) 9, 24, 60–61, 79, 82–83, 121
SHBG, see Sex hormone binding globulin
Sheehan's syndrome 59, 65, 94
Somatastin 3, 7

Spermatogenesis 11, 92
Spironolactone 83, 90
Sterilisation 68
Steroidogenesis 6, 10–11, 27–31, 37, 109
Supraoptic nuclea 1–2, 7

T4, see Thyroxine
Tamoxifen 97, 125
Tanycyte 1–2
Testes 10–11
Testicular feminisation syndrome 50–52, 57–58
Testosterone 4, 10, 15–17, 21–24, 29, 63, 79, 82, 111, 124
TFTs, see Thyroid function tests
Thelarche 43
Thromboxane 19
Thyroid 12
Thyroid function tests 33, 55, 63, 71, 82, 95, 117
Thyroid stimulating hormone 3–7, 12, 19, 32–33, 55
Thyrotoxicosis, see Hyperthyroidism
Thyrotrophin releasing hormone 3–4, 7, 32–33
Thyrotrophin releasing test 33, 36
Thyroxine (T4) 12–13, 32, 121
Thyroxine binding globulin 12, 121
Thyroxine binding prealbumin 12
Toxaplasmosis 98
Tri-iodothyronine 12–13
Triphasic pill 101, 103
TSH, see Thyroid stimulating hormone
Turner's syndrome 50, 52, 57

Ultrasound imaging 34, 38, 48–49, 51, 58, 60, 62–63, 94, 97, 103

Vaginitis, atrophic 115,

117, 122
Vasoactive intestinal
 protein 6–7
Vasopressin 7–8
Ventromedial nuclei 1–2
VIP, see Vasoactive
 intestinal protein
Virilization, see
 Hirsutism
Vitamin B6, see Pyridoxine

Weight loss related
 amenorrhoea 48, 58,
 63, 65–66, 93

X-rays 34, 51, 55

Zinc 88
Zona facticulata 15–16
Zona glomerulosa 15–16
Zona reticularis 15–16